NHA

PHLEBOTOMY STUDY GUIDE

2024-2025

*Conquer the CPT Certification
with Flying Colors!*

Q&A | Test | Extra Content

Robert Cliven

EXLUSIVE EXTRA CONTENTS FOR YOU IN THE LAST CHAPTER!

I have recently decided to give **gifts** to all our readers. Yes, I want to provide you with the assistance that will help you with your study you will receive:

- **MP3 audio files** ready to rock on your drive, at the gym, wherever you choose!
- **A digital copy** of this book, always at your fingertips.
- **A glossary** of critical terms to review wherever, whenever.
- **20 case studies** that put you right into the action!
- A PDF copy of the book **"Medical Terms for Healthcare Professions"**, your essential sidekick.
- **+600 flashcards <u>with pictures</u>** to maximize your learning and cut down your study time!

Extra content for you

FLASHCARDS
with picture!

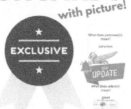

Extra content for you

CASE STUDIES

Extra content for you

AUDIOBOOK

You can track your progress and conveniently and interactively memorize the most important terms and concepts! Learn with printable flashcards or interactive flashcards on your device with **Anki APP or AnkiDroid!**

TABLE OF CONTENTS

INTRODUCTION

Embarking on a journey to becoming a certified phlebotomist opens up a world filled with profound knowledge and vital skills necessary to excel in the healthcare industry. This first chapter introduces the National Health career Association (NHA) Phlebotomy Exam Study Guide. As we progress, it will unfold as an essential companion that will help you navigate the comprehensive nature of this certification exam successfully.

The NHA is a renowned body that certifies various health professionals, including phlebotomists. The organization's core mission is to enable allied health professionals to expand their career opportunities. By taking this exam, you're on the path to enhancing your professional development, amplifying your skillset, and propelling your healthcare career to new heights.

The NHA Phlebotomy Exam, or the Certified Phlebotomy Technician (CPT) Exam, validates your competence as a phlebotomist. It examines your understanding of the knowledge and skills required to perform venipuncture and other related procedures. These include maintaining patient safety, effectively managing specimen collection, and demonstrating professional and ethical conduct.

Our study guide's primary objective is to streamline your preparation process by covering all topics in the NHA Phlebotomy Exam. We'll delve into areas such as infection control, legal issues in healthcare, phlebotomy procedures, and more. Each section will be clearly explained, with key concepts highlighted to ensure you fully grasp what to expect during the exam.

This guide also includes practical strategies for studying and test-taking, reinforcing your preparedness for the exam. We understand that everyone has a unique learning style. This guide offers varied techniques to cater to different learning preferences, from visual learners to those who prefer learning through practice.

Furthermore, this study guide contains several practice questions modeled after the actual exam's format, allowing you to gauge your understanding and readiness. The practice questions will be accompanied by detailed explanations to deepen your knowledge and clarify any areas of uncertainty.

By dedicating yourself to this study guide, you are not merely preparing for an exam. You are building a foundation of knowledge and skills to aid your professional journey as a phlebotomist. This guide serves as an invaluable resource, not only for the certification exam but for the rest of your phlebotomy career.

In this venture, every step you take brings you closer to the confident, competent, and certified phlebotomist you aspire to be. Remember, your commitment and determination are the keys to success. Let this NHA Phlebotomy Exam Study Guide be your roadmap to a promising and fulfilling career in healthcare. Welcome aboard!

Overview of the NHA Phlebotomy Exam

The Certified Phlebotomy Technician (CPT) Exam, administered by the National Health career Association (NHA), comprehensively evaluates the practical and theoretical knowledge necessary to excel in phlebotomy. It comprises 120 multiple-choice questions and delves into five key domains of phlebotomy.

- **Safety and Compliance:** This section focuses on vital concepts relating to maintaining a safe and compliant environment. It includes infection control, standard precautions, exposure control plans, and safety equipment and procedures.

- **Patient Preparation:** In this domain, you will be tested on understanding the steps necessary to prepare patients for phlebotomy procedures. Topics covered include patient identification, venipuncture site selection, communication, and interaction.

- **Routine Blood Collections:** This section dives into the primary skill of a phlebotomist, collecting blood samples. It tests your knowledge of various types of blood collection tubes, draw order, venipuncture technique, and post-venipuncture care.

- **Special Collections:** In this domain, the exam will assess your understanding of special collection procedures, including arterial blood gas collection, blood cultures, and collections from newborns and pediatric patients.

- **Processing:** The final section covers the processing and handling of collected specimens, including labeling requirements, proper transportation and storage methods, and procedures for dealing with rejected samples.

- **Specific eligibility criteria must be met to sit for the NHA Phlebotomy Exam.** This includes the successful completion of a training program or equivalent work experience. Specifically, candidates must complete a phlebotomy training program from an accredited institution within the last five years or have at least one year of supervised work experience as a phlebotomy technician practitioner within five years. Alternatively, candidates who've successfully performed several venipunctures and capillary sticks on live individuals may also be eligible.

This NHA Phlebotomy Exam is designed to thoroughly test your skills, knowledge, and abilities related to phlebotomy. Walking through each section of our study guide will prepare you for each domain and the questions you will encounter on the exam. Remember, your journey through this guide is an investment into your future as a certified phlebotomist. Let's venture forth and prepare you for your exciting career ahead!

PHLEBOTOMY BASICS

A critical first step to a rewarding career in phlebotomy is to comprehend the fundamentals of the profession. Phlebotomy is a complex process that requires rigorous technique, an understanding of anatomy and physiology, and superior patient care abilities. It involves more than merely extracting blood. The foundational concepts of phlebotomy will be covered in this chapter, establishing the platform for more complex subjects.

Understanding Phlebotomy

Blood is taken from patients during phlebotomy treatments for testing, donations, or medical procedures. You play a crucial part in the healthcare team as a phlebotomist. You frequently serve as the conduit between the patient and the lab, ensuring samples are adequately obtained and processed for appropriate test findings.

Roles and Responsibilities of a Phlebotomist

In addition to drawing blood, phlebotomists do other duties. They are accountable for accurately classifying patients, clarifying processes to ease patients' worries, choosing the right tools, performing venipunctures and capillary punctures, and ensuring the collected samples are correctly labeled and sent to the lab. Additionally, they must follow safety regulations to avoid cross-contamination and guarantee their and their patients' safety.

Anatomy and Physiology

Phlebotomy requires a thorough understanding of human anatomy, particularly the circulatory system. This information helps select the right veins for venipuncture, comprehend blood flow, and identify potential issues.

Types of Blood Draws

Depending on the patient's age, health, and the type of test requested, phlebotomists use various blood collection techniques. The two most used techniques are capillary puncture, sometimes known as a "finger stick," commonly used for little blood or when venous access is challenging. Venipuncture involves drawing blood from a vein, usually in the arm.

Equipment

It's essential to become familiar with the equipment needed for phlebotomy. These include sharps disposal containers, tourniquets, alcohol swabs, blood collection tubes, and personal protective equipment. Each piece of equipment is essential to the operation and helps to guarantee that it is done safely and correctly.

Patient Care

Providing top-notch patient care is the foundation of phlebotomy. Interacting with patients who could be uneasy or apprehensive is a common task for phlebotomists. Making the process as stress-free as feasible requires giving precise explanations, maintaining composure, and displaying empathy and understanding.

The following chapters will detail each of these fundamentals, examining their functions and how they work together to make phlebotomy practice effective and secure. The more thoroughly you understand these fundamental concepts, the more prepared you'll be to handle the profession's more complex facets.

Definition and Purpose of Phlebotomy

Phlebotomy, which derives from the Greek words "phlebos," which means "vein," and "tome," which means "to cut," focuses on the procedure of removing blood from the body. Contrary to its name, phlebotomy primarily entails poking holes in capillaries or veins (venipuncture or capillary puncture).

A phlebotomist or phlebotomy technician is a specialist who has received training and certification in this industry. These people are employed in various healthcare facilities, such as hospitals, diagnostic labs, blood donation facilities, and outpatient clinics. They are adept at numerous blood collection methods, ensuring patients have minor pain while receiving samples of the highest caliber for precise diagnosis and treatment.

Purpose of phlebotomy

Phlebotomy is essential to several aspects of healthcare, each of which emphasizes how important it is:

- **Blood draws are most frequently performed to help diagnose various medical disorders.** Laboratory findings are an essential source of information for doctors and other healthcare professionals when making decisions. Phlebotomists offer multiple tests to identify diseases, gauge organ function, evaluate nutritional condition, and more by taking blood samples.

- **Blood tests are essential for monitoring the effectiveness of medicines and managing chronic conditions.** Regular blood tests can determine whether a treatment works or changes are required. This includes keeping track of drug dosages in patients with illnesses like epilepsy, bipolar disorder, or organ transplants to check for potential toxicity or efficacy.

- **Routine blood tests are included in many preventative care programs.** Before symptoms even arise, these tests can help identify risk factors and early illness indicators, enabling early intervention and better health outcomes.

- **Phlebotomists play a crucial role in the blood donation industry.** They collect blood from donors to provide transfusions for patients who have lost blood through trauma, surgery, or illnesses like anemia. The safety of the blood obtained for the recipient as well as the safety of the donor, are ensured by phlebotomists.

- **Therapeutic phlebotomy:** Patients with certain disorders, such as hemochromatosis or polycythemia vera, may have excess iron or blood cells. The excess is eliminated, and these problems are managed with therapeutic phlebotomy. To prevent complications, phlebotomists skilled in this treatment must closely watch patients.

The significance of a phlebotomist's position within the healthcare team is highlighted by understanding the objective of phlebotomy. Their job directly affects patient diagnosis, treatment, and general health, emphasizing the significance of appropriate phlebotomy training and expertise. The vast importance of this profession on patient care and healthcare outcomes becomes even more apparent when we go deeper into the fundamentals of phlebotomy.

Responsibilities and Duties of a Phlebotomist

A phlebotomist is a crucial contributor to the healthcare ecosystem. Despite the primary duty of drawing blood, their responsibilities span a broader spectrum. This section elaborates on the multi-faceted role of a phlebotomist, including technical responsibilities and patient-centered duties, offering an in-depth understanding of aspiring phlebotomists.

Patient Identification and Preparation

Correct patient identification forms the foundation of the phlebotomist's duties. Phlebotomists must correctly identify the patient using at least two unique identifiers - typically the patient's name and date of birth. Ensuring accurate identification prevents severe medical errors, safeguarding the patient and healthcare providers.

Preparation extends to the patients, who must be adequately informed about the procedure to ensure their comfort and cooperation. This includes explaining the process, answering their questions, and assessing their physical condition for possible complications. For patients with physical disabilities or feeling unwell, phlebotomists may need to assist in positioning to facilitate a compelling blood draw.

Venipuncture and Capillary Puncture

The technical expertise of a phlebotomist is most evident in performing venipuncture and capillary puncture. Phlebotomists must master the correct procedure, including selecting the appropriate equipment, identifying the ideal puncture site, applying a tourniquet, and executing the puncture with minimal discomfort to the patient. They must handle different patient populations, including children, elderly individuals, and those with difficult venous access.

Specimen Handling and Processing

Post-draw, appropriate specimen handling, and processing are paramount. The phlebotomist must accurately label the sample, ensuring all information corresponds to the patient's details. They must also adhere to the correct storage and transport protocols for different types of specimens to maintain the sample's integrity. Phlebotomists may be involved in preliminary sample processing tasks like centrifugation in some healthcare settings.

Infection Control and Safety Measures

A phlebotomist is entrusted with maintaining a safe environment by adhering to strict infection control measures. This includes appropriate use of personal protective equipment (PPE), adherence to hand hygiene protocols, and safe disposal of sharps and other biohazardous waste. They must also be vigilant about potential hazards in the work environment and take immediate corrective measures.

Record Keeping

Accurate record-keeping is a fundamental duty of a phlebotomist. Records related to the blood draw must be meticulously documented, including the patient's information, the time and date of the procedure, and any issues or complications. These records are pivotal for quality control, auditing, and ensuring continuity and coordination of patient care.

Patient Communication

A phlebotomist's role extends beyond clinical tasks to include effective patient communication. Phlebotomists are often the first point of contact for patients and must provide clear explanations, answer queries, and offer reassurance to anxious patients. Mastery of active listening is essential to accurately interpret any concerns and respond empathetically to verbal and non-verbal cues from patients.

Team Collaboration

A phlebotomist's role doesn't exist in isolation; they are part of a broader healthcare team and must communicate effectively with other professionals. This could include promptly reporting unusual findings to a nurse or physician, collaborating with lab technicians about specific specimen requirements, or coordinating with administrative staff for accurate and timely patient records.

To summarize, a phlebotomist's role blends technical acumen, meticulous attention to detail, and a high level of patient interaction. While the responsibilities are multi-faceted, they offer a chance to impact patient care significantly. For individuals who enjoy working with people and contributing directly to healthcare outcomes, a career in phlebotomy can be gratifying. This complex role calls for a solid educational foundation and ongoing learning to stay abreast of the latest advancements in the field.

Ethical and Legal Standards in Phlebotomy

Ethical Standards

Ethical standards in phlebotomy form the bedrock upon which safe and effective patient care is built. Adhering to these guidelines ensures the phlebotomist's actions align with the healthcare professional's values. This section discusses the critical ethical standards in phlebotomy.

Patient Rights

Respect for patient rights is paramount in phlebotomy. Before consenting, patients have the right to be informed about any procedure, including the risks and benefits. They also have the right to refuse an approach. A phlebotomist must respect these rights, prioritizing open communication and shared decision-making with patients.

Confidentiality and Privacy

Phlebotomists handle sensitive patient data, such as medical histories, diagnoses, and test results. As per the Health Insurance Portability and Accountability Act (HIPAA), they must ensure the confidentiality of this information. They must also respect patients' privacy during procedures, such as by providing doors or curtains that are closed during a blood draw.

Professional Competence

Phlebotomists are ethically obligated to maintain competence and continually upgrade their skills and knowledge. They must only perform procedures they are trained and qualified to carry out. If a phlebotomist is unsure about a system, they should seek assistance rather than risk patient safety.

Non-maleficence

Non-maleficence, or 'not harm,' is a fundamental ethical principle. Phlebotomists must always prioritize patient safety, taking precautions to prevent harm. For instance, they should use the least invasive method possible for blood draws and adhere to infection control practices.

Quality Assurance

Phlebotomists play a crucial role in ensuring the quality of test results by following appropriate blood draw and specimen handling procedures. Mistakes in these processes can lead to inaccurate test results, affecting patient care. Phlebotomists have an ethical duty to prevent such errors and to report any issues that could impact quality.

Honesty and Integrity

Phlebotomists must uphold honesty and integrity, being truthful in their interactions with patients, colleagues, and other healthcare providers. This includes acknowledging mistakes and taking responsibility for them.

Respect for Colleagues

Phlebotomists should treat each other respectfully and professionally because they work as a team. This includes appreciating variety, working along with others, and resolving disagreements in a positive way.

Finally, upholding moral principles is essential to the phlebotomy profession. It generates a healthy work environment, builds trust between phlebotomists and patients, and ultimately helps provide high-quality patient care. In the following sections, we'll go into more detail about how these moral guidelines are put into practice in the course of regular phlebotomy practice.

Legal Standards

Like all medical specialties, phlebotomy operates within a set of rules and regulations intended to safeguard patients and healthcare professionals. Every phlebotomist must be aware of these legal requirements to ensure that their care falls within the bounds of the law. Let's examine these laws in greater depth.

Informed Consent

Informed consent is one of healthcare's most important legal concepts, including phlebotomy. According to this idea, a patient must know the procedure's goal, its risks and advantages, and any available alternatives before a phlebotomist can take their blood. The phlebotomist should record this consent procedure in the patient's medical file.

Patient Confidentiality

The Health Insurance Portability and Accountability Act (HIPAA) mandates that healthcare professionals, including phlebotomists, must preserve patients' private and medical information and uphold patient confidentiality. Phlebotomists must handle patient records securely and ensure they only divulge information to those allowed to help with the patient's care.

Professional Liability

Legal action may be taken against phlebotomists for their conduct. A phlebotomist may be held accountable if their carelessness or wrongdoing hurts a patient. This idea emphasizes how crucial it is to adhere to procedures, stay within the bounds of accepted practice, and keep one's competence up to date through ongoing education.

Scope of Practice

The obligations and responsibilities a phlebotomist is legally permitted to carry out are specified under the scope of practice. Depending on the state's legislation and the person's training and certification, these can change. To stay out of trouble with the law and their profession, phlebotomists should always remain within their area of expertise.

Mandatory Reporting

Certain situations legally require phlebotomists to report information. This could include suspicions of abuse or neglect or certain infectious diseases. Phlebotomists should be familiar with their state's mandatory reporting laws.

Discrimination Laws

Federal laws such as the Civil Rights Act and the Americans with Disabilities Act prohibit discrimination based on race, color, religion, sex, or disability. Phlebotomists must provide equal care to all patients and respect their rights, regardless of their background or characteristics.

In conclusion, understanding and adhering to legal standards are fundamental for every phlebotomist. It ensures the provision of care that respects patient rights, protects privacy, and promotes the safe and competent practice. As a phlebotomist, you must stay updated with these legal standards and incorporate them into your daily routine to deliver lawful and ethical patient care.

ANATOMY AND PHYSIOLOGY

A firm grasp of anatomy and physiology is crucial for phlebotomists as it allows them to safely and effectively draw blood, understand bodily reactions, and communicate with other healthcare professionals. In this section, we'll delve into the critical aspects of anatomy and physiology that every phlebotomist should know.

The Circulatory System

For phlebotomists, the vascular system is of utmost importance. This system, which comprises the heart, blood arteries, and blood, gets oxygen, nutrition, and hormones to all of the body's cells. The muscular organ that pumps blood throughout the body is the heart. The left and right atria and the left and right ventricles make up its four chambers. Among blood vessels are capillaries, veins, and arteries. Veins return deoxygenated blood to the heart, whereas arteries transport oxygenated blood to the body. Small blood arteries called capillaries are where waste and nutrients are exchanged. The complex tissue known as blood is made up of platelets, which aid in blood clotting, white blood cells, which fight infection, and red blood cells, which deliver oxygen.

Veins for Venipuncture

Venipuncture specialists need to be conversant with the veins that are frequently used. The median cubital vein, cephalic vein, and basilic vein are three significant veins that may all be found in the antecubital region of the arm, which is the preferred location for venipuncture. The antecubital region's median cubital vein in the center is typically the most secure and comfortable for the patient. Due to its proximity to arteries and nerves, the basilic vein on the pinky finger side is utilized less commonly, and the cephalic vein on the thumb side is frequently the second choice.

Hemostasis

Another important physiological term is hemostasis, which is the procedure that stops bleeding. The three processes involved are vasoconstriction (narrowing of the blood vessel), platelet plug creation, and coagulation (formation of a fibrin clot). Phlebotomists can control potential issues like bleeding or bruising following a blood draw by being aware of this procedure.

Immune Response

Phlebotomists also benefit from having a rudimentary understanding of the immune response, especially when discussing specific blood tests with patients. The immune system defends the body against illness by locating and eliminating infections and cancerous cells. The innate immune system, which serves as our initial line of protection, and the adaptive immune system, which develops a persistent defense against particular infections, are its primary parts.

Organ Systems

While phlebotomists primarily focus on the circulatory system, having a fundamental understanding of the body's other organ systems is advantageous. The endocrine system, for instance, controls hormones, many of which can be detected through blood testing. Our kidneys and bladder filter our blood and expel waste through the renal system. To exchange carbon dioxide and oxygen, the circulatory system collaborates closely with the respiratory system, which comprises the lungs and airways.

In conclusion, phlebotomists can work more safely and proficiently with a strong understanding of anatomy and physiology. Understanding test results, managing problems, and communicating with patients and other healthcare professionals are all made easier with the help of this information. We'll delve into these subjects in more detail and go over how they directly apply to the phlebotomy field in the following parts.

Detailed Overview of the Circulatory System

The circulatory system, also known as the cardiovascular system, is fundamental to phlebotomy. It is responsible for circulating blood throughout the body, delivering essential nutrients and oxygen while removing waste products. A detailed understanding of this system is crucial for any aspiring phlebotomist.

The Heart

The heart, located in the thoracic cavity between the lungs, acts as the system's central pump. It has four chambers: two atria on top (right and left) and two ventricles below. The right side of the heart receives oxygen-poor blood from the body and pumps it to the lungs. The left side receives oxygen-rich blood from the lungs and pumps it to the body. Electrical signals from the sinoatrial node regulate the heart's rhythmic contractions, often termed the heart's natural pacemaker.

Blood Vessels

Blood vessels are the channels through which blood flows. There are three main types:

- **Arteries:** These large vessels carry oxygenated blood from the heart to the body's tissues. The largest artery, the aorta, extends directly from the spirit and branches into smaller arteries, arterioles, and eventually capillaries.
- **Veins:** These vessels carry deoxygenated blood back to the heart. They start as tiny venules, which converge into more prominent veins. The most extensive veins, the superior and inferior vena cava, return blood to the heart.
- **Capillaries:** These tiny, thin-walled vessels connect arterioles and venules. They facilitate the exchange of oxygen, nutrients, and waste products between the blood and the body's cells.

Blood Composition

Blood is composed of cells suspended in plasma, a yellowish fluid. About 55% of blood is plasma, which carries nutrients, hormones, and waste products. The remaining 45% consists of:

Red Blood Cells (Erythrocytes): These cells contain hemoglobin, a protein that binds oxygen. They carry oxygen from the lungs to the body's tissues.

White Blood Cells (Leukocytes): These cells are part of the immune system and protect the body against infections and diseases.

Platelets (Thrombocytes): These cell fragments are crucial for clotting, a process that stops bleeding from a wound or incision.

Venipuncture Sites

In phlebotomy, the primary sites for venipuncture are the superficial veins in the antecubital area of the forearm:

- **Median Cubital Vein:** The first choice due to its size and location away from major nerves and arteries.
- **Cephalic Vein:** The second choice, often more significant in obese patients but harder to locate.
- **Basilic Vein:** The third choice is typically avoided due to its proximity to the brachial artery and the median nerve.

Understanding the circulatory system, including the structure and function of the heart, blood vessels, and blood, is foundational for phlebotomists. It guides safe and effective venipuncture, helps understand test results, and enables clear communication with other healthcare professionals. In the following chapters, we will dive deeper into the skills and techniques essential for successful phlebotomy, all building upon this foundational knowledge.

Venipuncture: Locating Appropriate Veins

Venipuncture, the process of drawing blood from a vein, is a central skill for any phlebotomist. A critical step in this process is locating appropriate veins for a blood draw. This section will guide you through the process of identifying the best veins for venipuncture.

Understanding Venous Anatomy

The first step is to understand the venous anatomy of the arm. As previously mentioned, the antecubital fossa, located at the bend of the elbow, is the primary site for venipuncture. Here you'll find three veins: the median cubital, the cephalic, and the basilic veins.

The median cubital vein is the first choice for most phlebotomists as it's often the most prominent and has fewer large nerves nearby. The cephalic vein, found towards the outer edge of the arm, is the second choice, while the basilic vein, closer to the body and nearer to nerves and arteries, is usually the last resort.

Patient Assessment

When choosing a vein, assessing the patient's physical characteristics and medical history is crucial. Age, weight, medical history, and hydration can influence vein prominence and suitability for venipuncture. For example, in well-hydrated patients, veins are often plumper and easier to access, while in elderly patients, veins may be more fragile and prone to bruising.

Vein Palpation

Visual assessment of the veins is essential, but palpation (feeling with the fingers) can give a more accurate idea of vein size, depth, direction, and condition. Veins suitable for venipuncture should feel soft, bouncy, and round. Problematic or cord-like veins may be thrombosed (clotted) and should not be used.

Using a Tourniquet

A tourniquet is typically applied about 3-4 inches above the venipuncture site to increase venous filling, making the veins more visible and palpable. It should be tight enough to impede venous flow but not arterial flow. However, it should be left on for at most 1 minute to avoid hemoconcentration and potential changes in test results.

Alternative Sites

If veins in the antecubital area are not accessible, phlebotomists may use alternative sites. These include veins on the back of the hand or the wrist, typically smaller and more prone to discomfort during venipuncture. In some cases, such as with infants or elderly patients with problematic veins, heel sticks or finger sticks may be used.

Understanding how to locate appropriate veins for venipuncture is critical to ensuring a successful blood draw. This skill takes practice, and phlebotomists can improve their abilities over time with hands-on experience. Patient comfort and safety are paramount, so take your time to find the best vein for each patient. Upcoming chapters will further explore the techniques and best practices for performing venipuncture safely and effectively.

PHLEBOTOMY PROCEDURES

Phlebotomy is more than just drawing blood; it is a series of procedures carried out with utmost precision to ensure patient safety, the accuracy of results, and the effectiveness of the medical treatment. This chapter will provide an overview of the various phlebotomy procedures that every phlebotomist should be well-versed in.

Patient Identification

The first and foremost step in any phlebotomy procedure is correctly identifying the patient. This is usually done by asking the patient to state their full name and date of birth, then verifying this information with the identification band worn by the patient and the test requisition form. This step is crucial to avoid medical errors and ensure the right patient gets the proper tests.

Test Verification

Once the patient's identity is confirmed, the phlebotomist verifies the tests ordered by the physician. This helps the phlebotomist understand the type and number of tubes required, the need for special preparations (like fasting or specific timing), and whether standard venipuncture, capillary puncture, or a particular collection procedure is required.

Equipment Preparation

Based on the ordered tests, the phlebotomist then prepares all necessary equipment. This typically includes the selection of appropriate needles, tubes, tourniquets, alcohol pads, gauze, and bandages. Special equipment may also be required for some tests, such as a butterfly needle for small or fragile veins or a lancet for capillary punctures.

Patient Preparation

The phlebotomist should also prepare the patient by explaining the procedure, answering questions, and ensuring the patient is comfortable and ready. This is also when the phlebotomist would apply the tourniquet and locate the best vein for venipuncture.

Blood Collection

The blood collection is performed using a technique known as venipuncture or, in some cases, a capillary puncture (fingerstick or heel stick). The phlebotomist must follow a specific order of draw when multiple tubes are collected to prevent cross-contamination of additives between lines.

Post-Collection Process

After blood collection, the phlebotomist should carefully remove the needle, apply pressure to the site to stop bleeding, and then bandage the area. They must also ensure the collected specimens are correctly labeled with the patient's information, test information, and time and date of collection.

Finally, the phlebotomist must handle and transport the samples appropriately to maintain their integrity. Depending on the tests ordered, this may involve specific temperatures, light conditions, or transport times.

These basic phlebotomy procedures ensure a successful and safe blood collection process. A good phlebotomist is meticulous about every step, ensuring the comfort and safety of the patient, the accuracy of test results, and effective communication with the rest of the healthcare team. In the upcoming chapters, we will detail each of these procedures, providing you with the knowledge and skills you need to excel in your phlebotomy practice.

Phlebotomy Equipment and Supplies

The phlebotomy field requires specialized equipment and supplies to ensure safe, effective, and successful blood draws. Familiarity with these tools is essential for every phlebotomist. This section will examine the various equipment and supplies used in phlebotomy, their uses, and how to handle them.

Venipuncture Supplies

- **Needles:** The most commonly used needles in phlebotomy are multi-sample needles designed to fit into a needle holder and allow multiple tubes to be filled from a single venipuncture. They typically range in size from 20- to 23-gauge, with the smaller numbers indicating larger needle diameters. The choice of needle size depends on the patient's vein size and condition.
- **Needle Holders:** Also called tube holders, plastic devices hold the blood collection needle on one end and the collection tube on the other. They are designed to allow a secure grip during the venipuncture process.
- **Evacuated Collection Tubes:** These vacuum-sealed tubes draw a predetermined blood volume into the tube. They are color-coded based on the type of additive they contain, which may be anticoagulants, clot activators, or special additives for specific tests.
- **Tourniquets:** These engorge veins and make them easier to palpate and visualize. They should be placed 3 to 4 inches above the venipuncture site and should not be left on for more than 1 minute.

Safety Supplies

- **Gloves:** Gloves protect both the phlebotomist and the patient from bloodborne pathogens. They should be worn at all times during the blood collection process.
- **Alcohol Swabs:** These are used to clean the venipuncture site before needle insertion. It's essential to allow the alcohol to dry completely before proceeding with the venipuncture to prevent stinging and hemolysis (destruction of red blood cells).
- **Gauze Pads and Bandages:** Gauze applies pressure to the venipuncture site after needle removal to stop bleeding, while bandages or adhesive strips cover the puncture site.

Blood Transfer Devices and Syringes

- **Blood Transfer Devices:** These are used to transfer blood from a syringe to a blood collection tube. They are helpful when the usual evacuated tube system cannot be used, such as when a butterfly needle is used, or the patient's veins cannot tolerate the vacuum pull of an evacuated tube.
- **Syringes:** Syringes may be used instead of evacuated tubes for venipuncture in certain situations, such as when veins are fragile and might collapse under the vacuum of an evacuated tube. Syringes allow the phlebotomist to control the speed and pressure of blood draw manually.

Capillary Puncture Supplies

- **Lancets** are small, sterile devices used to puncture the skin in capillary blood collection (such as fingersticks or heel sticks).
- **Microcollection Tubes:** Also called capillary tubes, these are small plastic tubes used to collect the drops of blood obtained from a capillary puncture. Depending on the tests ordered, they may contain additives similar to venipuncture collection tubes.

Miscellaneous Supplies

- **Specimen Labels:** After collection, each blood specimen must be immediately labeled with the patient's identifying information, the date and time of supply, and the phlebotomist's initials.
- **Sharps Container:** Used needles, lancets, and other sharps should be immediately disposed of in a sharp plastic container that is puncture-proof, **leak-proof, and properly labeled.**
- **Lab Transport Bags:** These unique bags transport collected blood samples to the laboratory. They have a separate pocket for the requisition form to prevent contamination.
- **Blood Smear Slides and Slide Covers:** These are used to prepare blood smears for microscopic examination.

Knowledge of phlebotomy equipment and supplies is vital for every phlebotomist. Understanding each tool's use and proper handling ensures you can perform the phlebotomy procedures efficiently and safely. In the following chapters, we will delve deeper into venipuncture and capillary puncture techniques, providing you with the practical knowledge you need to use these tools effectively.

Venipuncture Techniques

In the realm of phlebotomy, venipuncture is the most commonly performed procedure. To effectively draw blood without causing undue discomfort to the patient, a phlebotomist must master various venipuncture techniques. In this section, we delve into the methods used in venipuncture, offering scenarios for context to provide a comprehensive understanding of these crucial procedures.

The Standard Venipuncture Technique: A Fundamental Skill for Phlebotomists

Standard venipuncture involves withdrawing blood from a vein in the antecubital fossa using a straight needle and evacuated collection tubes. This technique is commonly used in adult patients, providing ample samples for multiple tests. The step-by-step process includes the following:

- **Preparing the Equipment:** Gather the necessary supplies, including the correct collection tubes, needle and needle holder, tourniquet, alcohol swabs, gauze, and bandage.
- **Patient Identification and Preparation:** Confirm the patient's identity and explain the procedure. Position the patient appropriately, apply the tourniquet, and locate the best **vein for venipuncture.**
- **Venipuncture Procedure:** Cleanse the site with an alcohol swab, allow it to dry, then insert the needle at a 15-30 degree angle with the bevel up. Once blood flow is established, fill the collection tubes in the correct draw order.
- **Post-Venipuncture Care:** Remove the tourniquet and needle, apply pressure to stop bleeding, and bandage the site. Make sure to dispose of used sharps immediately in a sharps container.

Butterfly Needles: A Special Technique for Small or Fragile Veins

Butterfly needles, or winged infusion sets, are often used for venipuncture on patients with minor or fragile veins, like elderly patients or children. The procedure is similar to the standard venipuncture technique, but there are a few key differences:

- **Needle Selection and Handling:** Butterfly needles are smaller and allow more delicate control, but they require a blood transfer device or a syringe for collection as they cannot directly accommodate evacuated tubes.
- **Vein Puncture:** The insertion angle is shallower with a butterfly needle, typically around 5-15 degrees. Once the vein is punctured, blood appears in the flashback chamber, signaling it's time to begin a collection.

Dorsal Hand Venipuncture: An Alternative for Difficult Antecubital Veins

Sometimes, it's challenging to locate suitable veins in the antecubital area. In these cases, the dorsal hand venipuncture technique can be utilized.

- **Vein Location and Puncture:** Veins on the back of the hand are generally smaller and closer to the surface. Using a butterfly needle is usually the best choice for these veins.
- **Patient Comfort:** Puncturing hand veins can be more uncomfortable for the patient. It's essential to reassure the patient and use a gentle technique to minimize discomfort.

Syringe Draw: A Solution for Weak or Collapsing Veins

A syringe draw technique may be employed when a patient's veins are prone to collapsing under the vacuum pressure of an evacuated tube.

- **Blood Draw:** With the syringe draw, the phlebotomist manually controls the pressure and speed of the blood draw, minimizing the chance of vein collapse.
- **Blood Transfer:** Blood must be transferred to collection tubes using a blood transfer device after the draw. The phlebotomist must carefully manage this process to avoid needlestick injuries and maintain sample integrity.

The world of venipuncture is vast and diverse, requiring various techniques to accommodate each patient's unique needs. By mastering these techniques, a phlebotomist can ensure a successful blood draw while maximizing patient comfort and safety. With practice and experience, these techniques will become second nature, making you a proficient and confident phlebotomist.

Capillary Puncture Techniques

Capillary puncture, also known as a skin puncture or fingerstick, is an essential procedure in phlebotomy. This technique is commonly used for collecting smaller blood samples, for pediatric patients, or when venous access is difficult. In this chapter, we explore capillary puncture techniques in-depth, outlining the various methods used to ensure a thriving collection of capillary blood specimens.

Fingerstick Technique: The Common Choice for Adult Patients

The fingerstick technique is often the go-to for capillary punctures in adults and older children. The steps include:

- **Patient Preparation:** As always, begin by correctly identifying the patient, explaining the procedure, and assembling all necessary supplies, which include a lancet, alcohol swabs, gauze, bandage, and micro collection tubes or blood smear slides.
- **Site Selection and Preparation:** The ideal site for a fingerstick is the third (middle) or fourth (ring) finger of the non-dominant hand. The fingertip should be warm; if not, gently massage the finger to increase blood flow. Cleanse the puncture site with an alcohol swab and let it air dry.
- **Capillary Puncture:** Hold the patient's finger firmly, then puncture the skin on the side of the fingertip (avoiding the center where there are more nerve endings) using a lancet. The depth of the puncture should be 2.0 mm for adults.
- **Blood Collection:** Wipe away the first drop of blood, which may contain tissue fluid, then collect the following reductions in your micro collection tube or onto your blood smear slide. Avoid 'milking' the finger, which can lead to hemolysis or contamination with tissue fluid.

Heel Stick Technique: Primarily for Infants and Young Children

A heel stick is the preferred method for capillary puncture in infants and young children. The process is slightly different from the fingerstick technique:

- **Site Selection and Warming:** The lateral or medial plantar surfaces are the appropriate sites for a heel stick. It's crucial to warm the heel before the procedure (using a warm cloth or commercial heel warmer) to increase blood flow.
- **Puncture Depth:** Use a lancet to make the puncture, ensuring the cut isn't deeper than 2.0 mm to prevent injury to the heel bone, especially in premature infants with thinner heel pads.
- **Blood Collection:** Like the fingerstick technique, discard the first drop of blood and then collect the following slides in your micro-collection tubes.

Special Considerations for Capillary Puncture

- **Order of Draw:** Unlike venipuncture, the order of draw for capillary puncture begins with blood gasses, followed by EDTA specimens (like hematology tests), other additive tubes, and finally, serum tubes.
- **Hematocrit and Hemoglobin Considerations:** Capillary blood has a slightly higher hematocrit and hemoglobin level than venous blood. It's essential to consider this when interpreting results.
- **Sample Mixing:** Unlike venipuncture, where tubes are inverted to mix the sample, capillary tubes should be rotated to mix the model and avoid hemolysis.

Capillary puncture is critical for phlebotomists, mainly when dealing with specific patient groups. By mastering these techniques, you can ensure that even small blood samples are collected effectively, ensuring the accuracy of test results and the overall success of the diagnostic process.

Safety Precautions and Infection Control in Phlebotomy

A crucial aspect of phlebotomy revolves around maintaining a safe environment and stringent infection control. As a phlebotomist, you are responsible for ensuring the safety of your patients and your own. This chapter will explore safety precautions and infection control measures in detail, highlighting their importance in every phlebotomist's daily routine.

Personal Protective Equipment (PPE): Your First Line of Defense

Wearing appropriate Personal Protective Equipment (PPE) is fundamental to prevent exposure to bloodborne pathogens. PPE includes gloves, gowns, masks, and eye protection. Gloves must be worn during every patient interaction, and other PPE should be donned whenever splashes or droplets are at risk. Remembering that PPE should be removed carefully to avoid self-contamination and disposed of in designated containers is vital.

Hand Hygiene: The Simplest Yet Most Powerful Prevention Tool

Hand hygiene must be stressed more. It's the most straightforward yet most powerful tool for preventing the spread of infection. Hand hygiene should be performed before donning gloves, after removing gloves, between patient interactions, and whenever hands are visibly soiled. Washing with soap and water for at least 20 seconds or using an alcohol-based hand sanitizer when soap and water are unavailable are effective hand hygiene methods.

Safe Handling and Disposal of Sharps

Needlestick injuries are a significant hazard in phlebotomy. Safe handling includes never recapping used hands, disposing of used sharps immediately in a puncture-proof sharps container, and using safety-engineered devices whenever possible. If a needlestick injury occurs, following your facility's post-exposure protocol is crucial, which usually includes washing the area, reporting the incident, and medical evaluation.

Bloodborne Pathogens Standard and Exposure Control Plan

The Occupational Safety and Health Administration (OSHA) regulates workplace safety through the Bloodborne Pathogens Standard in the United States. This regulation requires employers to have an Exposure Control Plan, offer Hepatitis B vaccinations to employees, provide PPE, and offer post-exposure evaluation and follow-up. As a phlebotomist, you should know your employer's Exposure Control Plan and understand your rights and responsibilities under the Bloodborne Pathogens Standard.

Proper Cleaning and Disinfection Practices

Regular cleaning and disinfection of phlebotomy areas are vital to prevent the spread of infection. All surfaces should be cleaned at the beginning and end of each shift and anytime there's a spill or contamination. Use an EPA-registered disinfectant or a bleach solution and follow the manufacturer's instructions for contact time.

Isolation Precautions

Some patients have conditions that require special isolation precautions to prevent the spread of infection. There are three types of isolation precautions: Contact (for diseases spread by direct contact), Droplet (for infections spread by large respiratory droplets), and Airborne (for infections spread by tiny airborne particles). Each type of precaution requires different PPE and practices, so knowing which precautions are necessary before entering a patient's room is essential.

To illustrate the importance of these precautions, consider a scenario in a busy hospital setting. Suppose a phlebotomist neglects to change gloves between patients. In this case, the phlebotomist might unknowingly transfer MRSA (Methicillin-resistant Staphylococcus aureus), a type of bacteria resistant to many antibiotics, from one patient to another, leading to a severe and hard-to-treat infection in the second patient. This example underscores the importance of consistent adherence to safety precautions and infection control measures in phlebotomy.

In conclusion, safety precautions and infection control form the bedrock of safe and effective phlebotomy practice. By integrating these principles into your everyday routine, you can protect yourself, your patients, and your colleagues from the potential spread of infectious diseases.

SPECIMEN COLLECTION AND HANDLING IN PHLEBOTOMY

In the diagnostics world, a phlebotomist's role extends far beyond the initial blood draw. A critical part of the job is the proper collection and handling of specimens to ensure the accuracy of laboratory results. This involves understanding different types of models, their specific collection procedures, how they should be handled post-collection, and the conditions required for their transportation and storage.

This chapter delves into the importance of proper specimen collection and handling, highlighting the phlebotomist's pivotal role in the diagnostic process. From understanding the unique requirements of various blood tests to knowing the ideal conditions for sample preservation, this chapter will thoroughly understand these vital aspects of phlebotomy work.

Precisely handling and managing specimens can dramatically impact a patient's diagnostic journey. For a clinician, a lab report is more than just numbers on a page - it is a crucial tool that can guide diagnosis, dictate treatment options, and track the progress of disease management. A phlebotomist's ability to maintain the integrity of collected specimens is a cornerstone to generating accurate and reliable lab results, thus ensuring the highest quality of patient care.

Labeling and Managing Specimens - A Paramount Step in Phlebotomy

The importance of proper specimen labeling and management cannot be overstated in phlebotomy. Mislabeling or mishandling specimens can lead to severe patient diagnosis and treatment errors. This section provides a detailed guide to accurate specimen labeling and effective specimen management, emphasizing best practices to maintain specimen integrity and prevent mistakes.

Labeling Specimens: Ensuring Accuracy and Precision

Every specimen collected from a patient must be appropriately labeled to maintain its traceability. The label should be affixed to the specimen container (not the lid) immediately after collection while still in the patient's presence. This real-time labeling ensures that specimens are correctly identified and helps prevent mislabeling errors.

Typically, a specimen label should include the following information:

- **Patient Identification:** This is usually the patient's full name per the hospital or laboratory record. The patient's ID number or date of birth might also be used for additional identification.
- **Date and Time of Collection:** This information helps track the specimen's age and can be crucial for tests that depend on specific timing.
- **Phlebotomist's Initials:** These allow traceability to the person who collected the specimen, which can be critical in clarifying any discrepancies or issues that might arise later.
- **Specimen Type and Source:** This information is essential for non-blood specimens, such as urine or tissue samples.

Managing Specimens: Preserving Integrity and Preventing Degradation

Once the specimen has been collected and labeled, it should be appropriately managed to preserve its integrity and prevent degradation. This involves understanding the specific requirements of various models, such as their ideal storage temperature, light sensitivity, and whether they require any special handling. For instance:

- **Temperature Considerations:** Some specimens need to be chilled immediately after collection (like lactic acid or ammonia), while others need to remain at body temperature (like cold agglutinins).
- **Light Sensitivity:** Test specimens like bilirubin or porphyrins should be protected from light to prevent degradation.
- **Timeliness:** Some specimens, such as those for blood cultures or glucose testing, should be transported to the laboratory as soon as possible to ensure accurate results.

Special Considerations for Non-Blood Specimens

While blood is the most commonly collected specimen in phlebotomy, phlebotomists collect non-blood specimens, like urine, stool, or throat swabs. These specimens have unique labeling and management requirements, such as including the source of the model on the label and following specific collection and preservation procedures.

Specimen labeling and management are integral to a phlebotomist's duties. Each step, from printing the correct label to ensuring the specimen's proper storage and transportation, requires attention to detail and knowledge of the specific requirements of different tests.

To illustrate this point, consider an **example**: a phlebotomist collects a blood sample for a potassium test. If the phlebotomist neglects to keep the specimen at the correct temperature, the cells in the model might break down, releasing potassium into the serum and resulting in a falsely elevated potassium result. This could lead to the patient receiving unnecessary and potentially harmful treatment for hyperkalemia, a condition of high potassium levels. This example underscores phlebotomists' critical role in patient care and the importance of proper specimen labeling and management in ensuring accurate laboratory results.

Collecting Special Samples - Mastery in Phlebotomy

Phlebotomy involves collecting diverse specimens for various laboratory tests, each requiring special handling and processing protocols. This section delves into the collection of individual samples, such as those required for glucose and coagulation testing, along with an overview of other specialized groups in phlebotomy.

Glucose Testing: Timing

Blood glucose testing is a standard diagnostic tool used to diagnose and manage diabetes. The timing of sample collection relative to the patient's last meal is crucial in this test. Fasting blood glucose requires the patient to abstain from eating for at least 8 hours before the sample collection, while random blood glucose can be collected at any time. The specimen for glucose testing should be transported to the lab immediately or mixed with a glycolytic inhibitor to prevent glucose breakdown by blood cells.

Consider a patient who is being evaluated for diabetes. The physician requests a Fasting Blood Glucose test. The phlebotomist instructs the patient not to eat or drink anything except water for at least 8 hours before the test. On the test day, the phlebotomist carefully collects a blood sample, ensuring immediate transportation to the lab to prevent glucose breakdown, possibly leading to falsely low glucose levels.

Coagulation Testing: The Delicate Balance

Coagulation tests, like Prothrombin Time (PT) or Activated Partial Thromboplastin Time (APTT), assess the blood's ability to clot. These tests require collection in a tube containing a specific anticoagulant—sodium citrate. Filling the tube to the correct volume is vital to maintain the precise ratio of blood to anticoagulant. Any deviation can lead to inaccurate results, potentially affecting patient treatment. Once collected, these specimens should be gently mixed and transported to the lab as soon as possible to prevent clotting.

A patient on warfarin (an anticoagulant) therapy needs regular PT/INR tests to monitor the effectiveness of the treatment. In this case, the phlebotomist should use a light-blue top tube containing sodium citrate and fill it to the correct volume. If the tube is underfilled, the excess anticoagulant might falsely prolong the PT, leading the physician to believe the patient's blood is too thin and consequently reduce the warfarin dose, potentially increasing the clot risk.

Blood Cultures: Hunting for Microbes

Blood cultures are used to identify bacteria or fungi in the blood. Since these specimens require a sterile technique to prevent contamination, they are usually drawn first in multiple draws. Blood culture bottles are inoculated with the model at the bedside, and the bottles are then incubated in the laboratory to encourage microbial growth for identification.

A patient comes in with symptoms of sepsis—a severe response to bacteria or other germs. The doctor orders blood cultures to identify the infectious organism. The phlebotomist carefully cleans the patient's skin with an antimicrobial agent and then sterilely collects blood into the culture bottles. Any contamination could lead to the growth of bacteria that aren't actually in the patient's blood, resulting in a false-positive result and unnecessary antibiotic treatment.

Therapeutic Drug Monitoring and Toxicology Tests: Precision in Collection

Some tests monitor medication levels in the blood (like Digoxin or Lithium) or screen for drugs or toxins. The timing of collection relative to the patient's last dose of medication is critical for therapeutic drug monitoring. Toxicology specimens often require specific collection tubes and might need immediate chilling or another special handling.

A patient with bipolar disorder is being treated with lithium. The physician requests lithium level tests periodically to ensure the drug level in the patient's bloodstream is therapeutic but not toxic. The phlebotomist must draw the blood sample just before the patient's next dose of lithium. Removing the piece too soon after the last amount might falsely elevate the lithium level, potentially leading to an unnecessary reduction in the medication dose.

Arterial Blood Gases (ABGs): Expertise Required

Arterial Blood Gases (ABGs) measure oxygen and carbon dioxide levels in arterial blood and blood pH. This test requires arterial blood, most often drawn by a physician or a trained phlebotomist from the radial artery. The specimen should be analyzed immediately or stored on ice until it can be processed, as delays can lead to changes in blood gas levels.

A patient with severe chronic obstructive pulmonary disease (COPD) has difficulty breathing. The physician orders an ABG test to assess the patient's oxygen and carbon dioxide levels. This blood sample must be taken from an artery, usually by a trained specialist. The collected specimen must be promptly transported on ice and processed quickly to prevent changes in the measured blood gas levels.

Collecting unique samples in phlebotomy requires an understanding of the specific collection, handling, and processing requirements of each test. A phlebotomist's skill in these collections directly impacts the accuracy of the test results and, consequently, the quality of patient care.

PATIENT INTERACTIONS

Patient interaction is essential to a phlebotomist's duties, often defining the quality of the patient's experience. This chapter explores the critical components of successful patient interactions in phlebotomy, providing a comprehensive guide to establishing rapport, handling difficult situations, and maintaining professionalism throughout the process. As a phlebotomist, your first interaction with a patient sets the tone for the entire encounter. Approaching patients with respect, empathy, and confidence eases their anxieties and fosters a sense of trust and cooperation.

Effective Communication: Key to Patient Trust

Clear and effective communication is crucial when dealing with patients. Always introduce yourself, explain the procedure to the patient, and answer any questions they might have. This open dialogue helps alleviate fears and uncertainties about the process. Be mindful of using layperson's terms rather than medical jargon to ensure patients understand your explanations.

Demonstrating Empathy and Patience

Some patients may exhibit fear or anxiety about blood draws. Children, elderly individuals, or those fearing needles (trypanophobia) may need additional reassurance. Show empathy, understanding, and patience in these situations, taking the time to comfort the patient and move at a pace comfortable for them.

Maintaining Professionalism

A phlebotomist should always maintain a high level of professionalism. This includes respecting patient privacy by following HIPAA regulations, wearing appropriate attire, and conducting oneself in a manner that promotes confidence in your abilities. Always observe ethical boundaries and avoid inappropriate conversations or actions.

Identifying and Verifying Patient Identity

One of the critical responsibilities in patient interactions is correctly identifying the patient before proceeding with the blood draw. Follow the established protocols of your facility for patient identification, usually involving checking the patient's ID band and having the patient confirm their name and date of birth.

Handling Difficult Interactions

There may be situations where you encounter uncooperative or complex patients. In these scenarios, maintain your composure, and use practical communication skills to manage the situation. Do not hesitate to involve a supervisor or other healthcare personnel if necessary.

Post-Procedure Care

Once the procedure is complete, provide the patient with aftercare instructions. Inform them about any signs of complications they should watch for, like prolonged bleeding or developing a hematoma, and what steps they should take if these occur.

Remember, as a phlebotomist, you play an essential role in the patient's overall experience within the healthcare setting. Your ability to interact effectively with patients, show empathy, and communicate clearly can significantly impact their comfort levels and overall impression of care received. Therefore, mastering patient interactions is a valuable skill that every phlebotomist should cultivate.

Patient Communication Techniques

Clear, compassionate, and effective communication is at the heart of excellent patient care in phlebotomy. This section explores various communication techniques and their application in phlebotomy, with real-world examples to enhance understanding.

Active Listening

Active listening involves fully concentrating, understanding, and responding to a speaker. Phlebotomy could mean paying close attention to a patient's concerns about a blood draw or their medical history and addressing them directly.

Example: A patient expresses fear about the pain of a needle. The phlebotomist listens attentively, acknowledges the patient's anxiety, and then explains how they will use a smaller gauge needle and specific techniques to minimize discomfort.

Non-Verbal Communication

Non-verbal communication includes body language, facial expressions, gestures, and tone of voice. Phlebotomists should maintain eye contact with patients, use open body language, and keep a gentle, calm voice to help patients feel at ease.

Example: A phlebotomist maintains a warm smile and eye contact with a child who is anxious about a blood draw, uses a soft tone of voice, and adopts a relaxed posture to appear less intimidating.

Clear and Concise Explanation

Phlebotomists should explain procedures in a clear, concise manner using language that patients can understand. Avoiding medical jargon helps patients feel more informed and less anxious about what to expect.

Example: Rather than telling a patient that they are going to perform a "venipuncture," a phlebotomist explains, "I am going to gently insert a small needle into a vein in your arm to collect some blood."

Empathetic Response

Empathy involves understanding and sharing the feelings of others. Expressing sympathy can make patients feel heard and supported.

Example: If a patient is nervous, a phlebotomist might say, "I understand that this can be a little nerve-wracking. I'm here to ensure we get this done as comfortably and quickly as possible for you."

Open-Ended Questions

Using open-ended questions can encourage patients to express their feelings and provide more information, which can be particularly helpful if a patient is anxious or hesitant.

Example: Instead of asking a yes-or-no question like "Are you nervous?" a phlebotomist could say, "Can you tell me how you're feeling about this?"

Validation and Reassurance

Phlebotomists should validate patients' feelings and provide reassurance, especially when anxious or fearful.

Example: "It's normal to feel nervous about this, but I want to assure you that I'll do my best to make this as comfortable as possible for you."

Teach-Back Method

The teach-back method involves asking patients to repeat the information you gave them to confirm their understanding. This method is particularly effective when providing aftercare instructions.

Example: After explaining how to care for the puncture site post-blood draw, the phlebotomist asks, "Can you tell me what you'll do when you get home?"

Positive Language

Using positive language can help create a more comforting environment for the patient. It's crucial to assure the patient that they are in capable hands and that everything is proceeding as it should.

Example: Instead of saying, "Don't move," the phlebotomist could say, "Stay nice and still for me." The latter communicates the same information but with a more positive spin.

Reflective Listening

Reflective listening involves paraphrasing or repeating what the patient has said to confirm understanding and show the patient that they have been heard.

Example: If a patient mentions they have had bad experiences with blood draws, the phlebotomist might respond, "It sounds like you've had some tough experiences with this before. I'm sorry to hear that. Let's work together to make this one as easy as possible."

Cultural Sensitivity

Being aware of and respectful of your patients' cultural norms and values is a crucial part of effective communication. This might involve understanding cultural norms about eye contact, personal space, or the use of touch.

Example: In some cultures, direct eye contact can be perceived as confrontational or disrespectful. If a patient seems uncomfortable with direct eye contact, the phlebotomist can adjust their approach and communicate respect for the patient's cultural practices.

Building Rapport

Building rapport involves creating a sense of mutual trust and understanding. This can involve small talk or finding common interests to make the patient feel more at ease.

Example: The phlebotomist might comment on the weather, ask about the patient's day, or talk about a local event, all the while being mindful of the patient's responses and comfort level with the conversation.

Feedback Encouragement

Encourage patients to provide feedback about their comfort levels during the procedure. This allows for adjustments as needed and gives the patient a sense of control over the situation.

Example: The phlebotomist can say, "If you feel uncomfortable at any point or need a break, please let me know. Your comfort is important to me."

By employing these techniques, phlebotomists can enhance patient communication, improve the patient's experience, and foster a more caring and effective healthcare environment.

Handling Difficult or Anxious Patients

Navigating complex or anxious patient interactions is a common challenge in phlebotomy. This section provides a detailed exploration of the strategies for managing these situations, punctuated by real-world scenarios to enhance understanding.

Recognizing Anxiety and Fear

Before phlebotomists can address patient fears, they need to recognize them. Signs of anxiety may include trembling, sweating, rapid speech or silence, refusal to make eye contact or even outright rejection to proceed with the blood draw. Being attuned to these signs enables the phlebotomist to take immediate steps to reassure the patient.

Scenario: A patient arrives for a routine blood draw and appears visibly shaking. Instead of proceeding directly with the appeal, the phlebotomist acknowledges the patient's fear, saying, "I notice you seem a bit anxious. It's okay; many people feel this way. We will go through this process together, step by step."

Tailoring Communication Style

Phlebotomists should be versatile in their communication styles and be ready to adjust according to the patient's needs. Some patients may require a gentler, more patient approach, while others may respond better to a more direct, no-nonsense style.

Scenario: An anxious patient asks a plethora of questions, seeking reassurance. The phlebotomist adapts to a patient-centered approach, answering each question thoroughly, using calming language, and demonstrating each step before performing it.

Gradual Desensitization

Gradual desensitization can help ease anxiety. This involves exposing the patient to the fear-inducing situation in a controlled, gradual manner. It's about walking patients through the procedure slowly and allowing them to adjust at their own pace.

Scenario: For a patient with extreme fear, the phlebotomist shows the equipment first, allows them to touch the unopened needle, and explains the sensation they might feel during the blood draw. This slow exposure helps reduce the fear associated with the unknown.

Use of Distractions

Distraction can be an effective technique to manage anxiety, particularly for pediatric patients or those with a significant fear of needles. This can involve talking about a non-related subject, asking the patient to look away, or using a distraction device.

Scenario: While performing a blood draw on a young child, the phlebotomist engages the child in a conversation about their favorite superhero, directing their focus away from the blood draw process.

Involving Family or Support Persons

Having a familiar face nearby can have a calming effect. If a patient is incredibly anxious or complicated, consider involving a family member, friend, or another staff member to provide reassurance.

Scenario: An elderly patient with dementia becomes agitated during the blood draw. The phlebotomist respectfully asks the patient's daughter, who accompanied her to the appointment, to hold her hand and talk to her during the procedure.

Employing Relaxation Techniques

Guiding patients through simple relaxation techniques can help alleviate anxiety. Deep, controlled breathing, progressive muscle relaxation, or visualization can be effective.

Scenario: A phlebotomist instructs an anxious patient to take deep, slow breaths and imagine a peaceful place, like a beach or forest, to distract their mind from the blood draw.

Dealing with Aggressive or Disruptive Behavior

While most anxious patients are more likely to withdraw, some may react with aggression or disruptive behavior. In these cases, it's crucial to remain calm, communicate effectively, and seek assistance when necessary.

Scenario: A patient becomes verbally aggressive, claiming they've been waiting too long. The phlebotomist maintains a calm demeanor, validates the patient's feelings, and apologizes for the delay, assuring them they will be attended to shortly.

In all these scenarios, the primary goals are to ensure the patient's comfort, secure cooperation, and successfully collect the blood sample. The strategies and examples above guide phlebotomists to manage various challenging situations with patients while maintaining professionalism and empathy.

Providing Patient Care Post-Puncture

As integral as the pre-puncture and puncture phases are in phlebotomy, so is the post-puncture patient care. This stage allows phlebotomists to ensure the patient recovers seamlessly, mitigate potential complications, and enhance patient satisfaction. This section elaborates on several aspects of patient care after the venipuncture procedure.

Managing Immediate Aftercare

Once the blood sample has been obtained, the phlebotomist must immediately engage in aftercare. This involves promptly removing the needle, engaging the safety feature, and appropriately disposing it in a sharps container. Following this, applying firm pressure to the puncture site with a clean gauze or cotton ball is essential to stop bleeding.

Example: Consider an instance where a patient has a robust blood flow or is on blood-thinning medication. The phlebotomist may need to apply pressure to the puncture site for longer to ensure the bleeding has stopped entirely.

Application of a Dressing or Bandage

After ensuring the bleeding has ceased, the phlebotomist should apply a dressing or bandage to the puncture site. This helps protect the wound from external contaminants, preventing potential infection.

Example: A phlebotomist might need to explain why a bandage is necessary to a patient who dislikes wearing them. They could say, "This bandage will keep the site clean and help you avoid infection. It's best to leave it on for a few hours."

Providing Post-Puncture Instructions

Providing clear instructions for aftercare is crucial. Patients should be advised to leave the bandage on for a certain number of hours, avoid heavy lifting or strenuous activity with the punctured arm, and watch for signs of infection.

Example: In the case of a patient scheduled for several lab tests requiring fasting, the phlebotomist might advise, "Now that we've completed your blood draw, make sure to have a good meal and drink plenty of fluids."

Monitoring for Adverse Reactions

Phlebotomists should closely monitor patients for adverse reactions immediately after the procedure. While fainting, dizziness, or nausea are rare, they can occur, and the phlebotomist should be prepared to react accordingly.

Example: If a patient looks pale and sweaty after a blood draw, the phlebotomist should recognize these as signs of a potential fainting episode. Immediate action involves having the patient lie down and elevate their feet.

Offering Comfort and Reassurance

Continued reassurance and comfort post-puncture can be incredibly beneficial for the patient. This is especially true for anxious patients or those with a painful or difficult draw. The phlebotomist's words and actions can significantly impact the patient's overall experience.

Example: After a particularly challenging blood draw with a needle-phobic patient, the phlebotomist could provide comfort and praise, "You did well throughout that. It wasn't easy for you, but it's all done now. Take some time to relax and treat yourself today."

Documentation and Follow-ups

Finally, proper documentation is a crucial aspect of post-puncture care. The phlebotomist should update the patient's records with details of the procedure and any noteworthy occurrences. In case of any complications or issues, follow-up appointments might be needed.

Example: In a situation where a patient experiences an uncommon reaction, like prolonged bleeding, the phlebotomist should document this in the patient's records and inform their healthcare provider for potential follow-up.

By carefully managing these post-puncture care aspects, phlebotomists can significantly enhance the patient's overall experience, ensuring their health, safety, and satisfaction with the care received.

FAQS

How does the NHA Phlebotomy Exam work?
The Phlebotomy Technician Certification (CPT) exam from the National Health career Association (NHA) is a widely respected certification test. The exam aims to determine whether aspirant phlebotomists are qualified and prepared for the field and whether they meet the minimum requirements for education and experience.

2. What steps must I take to qualify for the NHA Phlebotomy exam?
Phlebotomy training programs and one year of supervised work experience as a phlebotomy technician are both required for eligibility to take the NHA Phlebotomy exam. You also need to possess a high school diploma or its equivalent.

3. How many questions, and what are the main sections, are there on the NHA Phlebotomy Exam?
There are 120 questions in the NHA Phlebotomy exam. Safety and compliance (20%), Patient Preparation (20%), Routine Blood Collections (40%), Special Collections (10%), and Processing (10%) comprise the five portions of the exam.

4. What kind of preparation should I do for the NHA Phlebotomy exam?
All subjects covered in your phlebotomy training program should be thoroughly reviewed to prepare for the NHA Phlebotomy exam. Study aids and practice exams are both beneficial resources. Additionally, you should review the anatomy and physiology of the circulatory system, phlebotomy techniques, patient relations, and laboratory safety regulations.

5. What is the NHA Phlebotomy Exam passing score?
A scaled scoring method is employed to obtain the passing result for the NHA Phlebotomy exam. The lowest passing score is 390, with a range of 200 to 500.

What occurs if I don't pass the NHA Phlebotomy exam?
You are permitted to repeat the NHA Phlebotomy exam if you fail it. However, there is a 30-day waiting period before you can retake the test.

7. If I fail the NHA Phlebotomy exam, how many may I repeat it?
The NHA Phlebotomy exam may be retaken as much as necessary to pass, but you must wait 30 days between each attempt. Please be aware that there is a new exam cost for each try.

8. How long does the NHA Phlebotomy Certification remain in effect?
For two years, the NHA Phlebotomy Certification is valid. Phlebotomists must fulfill continuing education requirements and pay a renewal fee to keep their certification.

9. Is the NHA Phlebotomy Exam available online?
No, to maintain the validity of the exam procedure, the NHA Phlebotomy exam must be taken in person at an authorized testing facility.

10. What is the registration process for the NHA Phlebotomy exam?
On the official website of the NHA, candidates can register online for the NHA Phlebotomy exam. You must first create an account to register for the exam, fill out the application, and pay the price.

What do I need to bring to the NHA Phlebotomy exam?
Bring a legitimate form of identification, such as a passport or driver's license. The name on the ID and the exam registration must be identical. You won't be permitted to bring personal goods into the testing area, including bags, books, phones, food, and drink.

What kinds of inquiries may I anticipate on the NHA Phlebotomy exam?
Multiple choice, drag and drop, and hotspot questions are among the question formats present on the NHA Phlebotomy exam. The questions will evaluate your understanding of phlebotomy practices, safety and compliance, patient preparation, regular and unique collections, and specimen processing.

13. When will I get the results of my NHA phlebotomy exam?
Most of the time, you'll get your results after passing the NHA Phlebotomy exam. According to the findings, your performance in each exam area will be broken down along with a breakdown of whether you passed or failed.

14. What are the advantages of NHA Phlebotomy Certification for My Career?
The achievement of an NHA Phlebotomy certification shows your dedication to professional growth and may improve your employment. It shows that you are proficient in phlebotomy at the level of nationally recognized standards, giving patients and employers alike peace of mind.

15. What occupations are available to me with an NHA Phlebotomy certification?
If you have an NHA Phlebotomy certification, you can work as a phlebotomy technician in various healthcare settings, including hospitals, diagnostic labs, blood donation facilities, and doctor's offices. Thanks to the certificate, you can be qualified for higher-level positions in laboratory services.

How can I keep my NHA phlebotomy certification current?
You must finish at least ten continuing education credits every two years and pay a recertification fee to keep your NHA phlebotomy certification current. The ongoing education needs to apply to phlebotomy.

17. Can people with impairments taking the NHA Phlebotomy exam receive accommodations?
In line with the Americans with Disabilities Act, NHA offers accommodations to people with verified disabilities. Accommodations can be requested throughout the exam application procedure.

18. May I change the date of my NHA Phlebotomy exam?
You may change the date of your NHA Phlebotomy exam, yes. You must book a new exam time at least 24 hours before the original, and rescheduling costs can be charged.

19. How should I prepare for the NHA Phlebotomy exam?
You should unwind the day before the test and avoid any last-minute studying. Make sure you are familiar with the testing site and exam timing. Get a good night's sleep and gather all of your exam-related supplies.

20. what subjects should I pay the most attention to
 for the NHA Phlebotomy exam?
While reviewing everything covered on the NHA Phlebotomy exam is crucial, pay close attention to the portions with the most questions. These include patient preparation, safety and compliance, and routine blood draws.

What should I bring on the day of the test?
- Attending an educational institution to take an online test: A current government-issued ID card, such as a driver's license or passport, is required. Any form of identification you present must match the name you used to register for the test.
- Testing with paper and pencil in a classroom: A current government-issued ID card, such as a driver's license or passport, is required. Also needed are two sharpened and prepared number-2 pencils.
- PSI Facilities for the Test: When you sign up for the exam, you can choose the authorized location where you will take it. Each site will require a government-issued photo ID before you can begin the exam as proof of identity.

QUESTIONS AND ANSWERS

Safety and Compliance

Adherence to Regulations such as OSHA, HIPPA, Operational Standards, Ethical Standards

What is the primary purpose of OSHA regulations in the healthcare setting?
The Occupational Safety and Health Administration (OSHA) sets guidelines to ensure safe and healthy working conditions. These regulations protect workers from hazards such as infections, harmful substances, and workplace injuries in healthcare.

How does HIPAA protect patient information?
The Health Insurance Portability and Accountability Act (HIPAA) safeguards individuals' medical information privacy. It restricts who can access or share a patient's protected health information (PHI) without explicit consent.

What are some common operational standards in a healthcare setting?
Operational standards vary across healthcare settings, but they often involve safety procedures, infection control protocols, patient confidentiality, and professional conduct.

Why are ethical standards necessary in healthcare?
Ethical standards guide healthcare professionals' behavior, promoting trust, respect, and fairness. They ensure patients' rights, protect their autonomy, and encourage the delivery of high-quality care.

What are the penalties for violating OSHA regulations?
Penalties can include hefty fines, mandatory corrective action, increased inspection rates, or even criminal charges in severe cases.

What information does HIPAA consider to be protected health information (PHI)?
PHI includes any health information that can be linked to a specific individual, including medical records, treatment history, billing information, and more.

How can healthcare professionals ensure they are adhering to operational standards?
Professionals can stay informed about current standards, attend continuous training, and implement checks and balances in their daily routines to maintain compliance.

Can you provide an example of an ethical dilemma in healthcare?
An example might be a patient refusing a lifesaving treatment due to personal beliefs. The healthcare provider must respect patients' autonomy while advocating for their health.

How does OSHA enforce safety standards in the workplace?
OSHA enforces safety standards through workplace inspections, response to employee complaints, and penalties for non-compliance.

What steps can healthcare organizations take to ensure compliance with HIPAA?
They can provide regular training, implement strict security measures for PHI, conduct periodic audits, and enforce disciplinary actions for non-compliance.

Quality Control

Why is quality control important in healthcare?
Quality control ensures consistency, accuracy, and reliability in healthcare services, directly affecting patient safety and treatment outcomes.

What is the role of a phlebotomist in quality control?
Phlebotomists ensure quality control by following proper blood collection procedures, correctly labeling specimens, and maintaining sterilization protocols to prevent cross-contamination.

Can you provide an example of a quality control procedure in a healthcare setting?
An example might be regularly calibrating laboratory equipment to ensure the accuracy of test results.

How does quality control affect patient care?
Quality control directly impacts patient care as it ensures accurate diagnoses and effective treatment plans, ultimately leading to better patient outcomes.

What are some standard quality control measures in phlebotomy?
These can include correctly identifying the patient, using proper venipuncture technique, adhering to the order of draw, ensuring correct labeling and storage of samples, and maintaining cleanliness.

What are the consequences of poor quality control in healthcare?
Poor quality control can lead to diagnostic errors, ineffective treatments, increased healthcare costs, and may jeopardize patient safety.

How can healthcare professionals ensure quality control?
They can regularly review and update protocols, participate in continuous training, and adhere to best practices in their field.

What is the role of continuous improvement in quality control?
Continuous improvement allows for constantly evolving quality control measures based on new information, feedback, and changing standards, ensuring that healthcare delivery remains practical and up-to-date.

Sharps Disposal

What is the proper procedure for disposing of sharps in a healthcare setting?
Sharps should be immediately placed in an FDA-cleared, puncture-resistant sharps disposal container. These containers should be easily accessible, maintained upright, and replaced promptly when they become three-quarters full.

Why is proper sharps disposal important?
Proper sharps disposal is crucial for preventing accidental injuries and potential transmission of bloodborne pathogens, such as HIV, Hepatitis B, and Hepatitis C.

What should healthcare workers do if they suffer a needlestick injury?
They should immediately wash the area with soap and water, report the incident to their supervisor, and seek immediate medical attention for further evaluation and treatment.

What should I do if the sharps disposal container is full?
A full sharps container should always be well-filled. It should be securely closed and then placed in a secondary container if leakage is possible. The entire container should be disposed of following the facility's policy and state regulations.

Can sharps be disposed of in regular trash?
No, sharps should never be disposed of in regular trash or recycling. They should only be placed in appropriate sharps disposal containers.

What types of items are considered sharps?
Sharps include any objects that can pierce the skin, including needles, scalpels, lancets, broken glass, and even exposed ends of dental wires.

What are the penalties for improper sharps disposal?
Penalties can range from fines to imprisonment, depending on the severity of the violation and the local regulations.

What should I do if I come across improperly disposed sharps?
Never handle sharps directly. Use a tool to pick them up, such as tongs or forceps, and place them in a sharps disposal container. Report the situation to the appropriate supervisor.

How can healthcare facilities prevent improper sharps disposal?
They can provide frequent training on sharps safety, make sharps disposal containers easily accessible, regularly audit disposal practices, and enforce strict penalties for non-compliance.

Can sharps disposal containers be reused?
No, FDA-cleared sharps disposal containers are single-use items and should not be opened, emptied, or reused.

Personal Protective Equipment (PPE)

Why is PPE essential in healthcare?
PPE is a physical barrier between healthcare workers and environmental hazards, including infectious diseases, chemicals, and bodily fluids, protecting them from potential harm.

What are some examples of PPE used in healthcare?
PPE includes gloves, gowns, masks, respirators, face shields, and eye protection.

What is the correct order for putting on and taking off PPE?
The order for donning PPE is a gown, mask/respirator, goggles/face shield, and gloves. The demand for doffing is gloves, goggles/face shields, gowns, and masks/respirators.

How often should PPE be replaced?
PPE should be replaced between patient encounters and whenever it becomes soiled or damaged.

What is the proper way to dispose of PPE?
Most PPE is disposable and should be thrown away in a designated receptacle. Some PPE, like goggles or face shields, can be disinfected and reused per facility policy.

What happens if PPE needs to be used correctly?
Incorrect use of PPE can expose healthcare workers to potential harm, including infections and chemical injuries.

Can I wear the same gloves for different patients if I sanitize them in between?
No, gloves should be changed between patients to prevent cross-contamination.

What should I do if my PPE becomes damaged during use?
Damaged PPE should be removed and replaced immediately to maintain protection.

Are there different types of masks for different situations?
Yes, surgical masks protect against large droplets, while N95 respirators provide a higher level of protection by filtering out smaller particles.

What is the role of respirators in PPE?
Respirators, such as N95 masks, protect healthcare workers from inhaling small airborne particles, including infectious agents.

Patient Preparation

Receiving Consent

What is the proper way to document patient consent in phlebotomy?
The consent process should be documented in the patient's medical records, including the information provided, the patient's capacity to understand, and their explicit agreement to the procedure. Some institutions also require a signed consent form for specific functions.

Can a patient withdraw their consent during a phlebotomy procedure?
A patient can withdraw their consent at any point during the phlebotomy procedure. If this happens, the procedure must be stopped immediately, and the situation should be discussed with the patient and their healthcare provider.

How can phlebotomists ensure that they have obtained informed consent?
Informed consent can be confirmed by giving the patient all necessary information about the procedure, checking their understanding, allowing them to ask questions, and getting their voluntary agreement to proceed.

What if a patient is incapable of giving consent?
If a patient cannot consent, a legal guardian or designated healthcare proxy can provide consent, following specific legal guidelines.

Identifying Special Considerations

How should phlebotomists handle patients with needle phobia?
For patients with needle phobia, use a gentle and empathetic approach, explain the procedure, employ distraction techniques, and, if possible, use smaller gauge needles.

What special considerations are needed for geriatric patients?
Geriatric patients may require special care due to fragile veins, potential cognitive issues, or chronic conditions. Patience, effective communication, and a gentle technique are key.

How do you handle blood collection from a patient with a mastectomy?
For mastectomy patients, avoid blood collection from the arm on the side of the surgery. This is to prevent the risk of lymphedema.

What should be done if a patient has a blood disorder such as hemophilia?
For patients with bleeding disorders like hemophilia, apply pressure to the venipuncture site for longer than usual after the draw and closely monitor the patient for signs of excessive bleeding.

How can you make a pediatric patient comfortable during a blood draw?
Use age-appropriate explanations, distraction techniques, a gentle approach, and smaller gauge needles for pediatric patients.

How should you handle a difficult venipuncture due to obesity?
In cases of obesity, use a longer and larger gauge needle. Also, a blood pressure cuff can be beneficial for locating deeper veins.

Interactions with Patients

What strategies can calm a nervous patient before a blood draw?
Active listening and empathy can help address a patient's concerns. Offering clear explanations about the procedure and maintaining a calm, confident demeanor can also help to ease their nerves.

How can you explain a delay in procedure to a patient who has been waiting for a long time?
Honest and respectful communication is critical. Apologize for the delay, provide a reasonable explanation without going into unnecessary details, and offer a revised timeline if possible.

How should a phlebotomist respond if a patient becomes angry or upset during a blood draw?
Maintain professional composure, listen to the patient's concerns without interruption, apologize if necessary, and offer to bring in a supervisor or doctor if the situation cannot be resolved.

How can phlebotomists ensure they respect a patient's privacy and confidentiality?
Discussing personal health information only in private, avoiding unnecessary exposure during the procedure, and following HIPAA guidelines are crucial steps in protecting patient privacy and confidentiality.

How do you establish trust with a patient you are meeting for the first time?
Start by introducing yourself and your role, explain the procedure clearly, answer any questions they might have, and maintain a respectful and empathetic demeanor throughout the interaction.

What is the importance of body language during patient interaction?
Positive body language, like maintaining eye contact and adopting an open posture, can help build trust and rapport with the patient. It can convey empathy, attentiveness, and respect.

Routine Blood Collection

Equipment Assembly

What are the main pieces of equipment needed for a routine venipuncture?
The main pieces of equipment include a tourniquet, alcohol wipes for antiseptic, disposable gloves, a blood collection device such as a syringe or evacuated tube system, and blood collection tubes.

Why is it important to assemble all the necessary equipment before starting a venipuncture procedure?
Assembling all necessary equipment beforehand minimizes the need to leave the patient during the procedure, reduces the risk of errors, and ensures a smoother, more efficient process.

What considerations should be taken into account when choosing the appropriate needle for a venipuncture?
The needle size should be chosen based on the patient's vein size and condition. Generally, a smaller gauge needle is used for fragile or small veins.

When should a butterfly needle be used in phlebotomy?
A butterfly needle, also known as a winged infusion set, is often used for difficult draws, such as in elderly patients, children, or when veins are small, fragile, or hard to locate.

What steps can be taken to ensure that phlebotomy equipment is safe and clean?
Equipment should be kept in sealed packages until use and regularly inspected for damage, and any reusable equipment should be properly cleaned and sterilized according to the manufacturer's instructions and institutional policies.

Following Order of Draw in Venipuncture

Why is the order of draw important in phlebotomy?
Following the correct order of draw reduces the risk of cross-contamination between tubes and ensures the accuracy of test results.

What is the recommended order of draw in venipuncture?
The recommended order is blood culture bottles, coagulation tubes (light blue), serum tubes with or without clot activator (red, gold), heparin tubes (green), EDTA tubes (lavender), and glucose tubes (gray).

How can you remember the order of draw?
One method is to use a mnemonic like "Boys Love Ravens That Gather Bird Eggs," which stands for Blood cultures, Light Blue, Red, Tiger (Gold), Green, Blue (Royal), and Eggshell (Lavender).

What could happen if the order of draw needs to be followed correctly?
Incorrect order of draw can lead to cross-contamination between additives in different tubes, potentially causing inaccurate test results, which can affect patient diagnosis and treatment.

Can the draw order differ between using a syringe and an evacuated tube system?
The draw order is generally the same regardless of the blood collection system. The order is determined by the additive in the tube, not the collection system.

Applying Antiseptic Agent

Why is it essential to use an antiseptic agent before a venipuncture?
Applying an antiseptic agent reduces the number of microbes on the skin, decreasing the risk of infection.

How should an antiseptic agent be applied to the venipuncture site?
The antiseptic agent, usually 70% isopropyl alcohol, should be applied using a circular motion from the center of the draw site outward and allowed to air dry before the venipuncture is performed.

What should you do if a patient is allergic to the antiseptic agent you plan to use?
An alternative agent should be used if a patient is allergic to the planned antiseptic. Common alternatives include chlorhexidine gluconate and povidone-iodine.

Can the venipuncture site be palpated after the antiseptic agent has been applied?
Palpation of the venipuncture site after applying the antiseptic should be avoided as it can decontaminate the area. If necessary, a new location should be selected, and the antiseptic process should be repeated.

Is using an antiseptic agent necessary for fingerstick or heel stick procedures?
Yes, an antiseptic should also be used for skin puncture procedures to minimize the risk of infection.

Labeling

What information is required on a specimen label?
A specimen label should include the patient's full name, date of birth or other unique identifiers, date and time of collection, and the phlebotomist's initials.

When should specimens be labeled?
Specimens should be labeled immediately after collection, in the patient's presence, to minimize the risk of errors.

What could happen if a specimen is improperly labeled?
Improperly labeled specimens can lead to identification errors, potentially causing incorrect diagnosis and inappropriate treatment and compromising patient safety.

Can a phlebotomist correct a label if they notice a mistake after the patient has left?
If a mistake is noticed after the patient has left, the specimen is typically discarded, and a new sample is collected. Correcting a label outside the patient's presence is not recommended due to the risk of misidentification.

What should a phlebotomist do if a patient refuses to confirm their identity for specimen labeling?
If a patient refuses to confirm their identity, the phlebotomist should explain the importance of proper identification for the safety and accuracy of their test results. If the patient refuses, the phlebotomist should contact their supervisor for further instructions.

Post-procedure Care

What are the steps for post-procedure care after a venipuncture?
After venipuncture, the needle should be safely discarded in a sharps container, pressure applied to the puncture site, and a bandage applied once the bleeding has stopped. The patient should be observed for adverse reactions and advised about necessary aftercare.

How long should pressure be applied to a venipuncture site after needle removal?
Pressure should be applied to the venipuncture site for at least 2-3 minutes after needle removal or until bleeding has stopped. This time may need to be extended for patients with bleeding disorders.

What advice should be given to a patient after a venipuncture procedure?
Patients should be advised to keep the bandage on for a few hours, to avoid strenuous activity with the arm used for the draw, and to seek medical advice if they experience prolonged bleeding or bruising.

What should a phlebotomist do if a patient faints during or after a venipuncture?
If a patient faints, the procedure should be stopped immediately, ensuring the patient's safety. If the patient is seated, they should be helped to lie down. Medical assistance should be sought immediately.

What signs of a post-procedure infection should a patient be made aware of?
Patients should seek medical advice if they notice signs of infection such as redness, swelling, increased pain, discharge from the puncture site, or if they develop a fever.

Special Collection

Non-Blood Specimen

What are some examples of non-blood specimens that a phlebotomist may be asked to collect?
Some examples of non-blood specimens include urine, saliva, sputum, stool, and swabs from various sites (nasal, throat, wound, etc.). These specimens can provide valuable information about a patient's health status.

What is the recommended method for collecting a urine specimen?
The mid-stream clean-catch method is most commonly used for urine collection. It involves the patient cleaning the genital area, urinating, and then collecting the middle part of the urine stream in a sterile container.

What special instructions should a patient be given when collecting a stool sample?
Patients should be instructed not to contaminate the stool with urine or toilet paper and to avoid overfilling the container. If applicable, they should also be made aware of any dietary restrictions before the collection.

Why is it important to properly label a non-blood specimen?
Proper labeling is crucial for testing the correct patient's specimen, avoiding misdiagnosis or improper treatment. Labels typically include the patient's name, date of birth or other identifiers, date and time of collection, type of specimen, and collector's initials.

What are some considerations for handling and storing non-blood specimens?
Considerations include using appropriate containers, maintaining proper temperature (some may need refrigeration), and timely transport to the laboratory to ensure sample integrity.

Skin Preparation

Why is skin preparation essential before a venipuncture?
Skin preparation reduces the number of microbes at the puncture site, decreasing the risk of contamination of the specimen and local infection.

What agent is most commonly used for skin preparation in routine venipuncture?
The most commonly used agent is 70% isopropyl alcohol due to its quick action and effectiveness against various microorganisms.

How should the antiseptic agent be applied to the skin?
The antiseptic should be applied circularly from the center of the puncture site outward and allowed to air dry.

Can the venipuncture site be touched after the antiseptic has been applied?
After the antiseptic has been applied and allowed to dry, the puncture site should not be touched. The site should be re-cleaned with antiseptic if it's connected or palpated.

What should you do if a patient is allergic to the antiseptic agent?
An alternative should be used if a patient is allergic to the standard antiseptic agent. For example, if the patient is allergic to iodine-based solutions, an alcohol or chlorhexidine-based antiseptic could be used instead.

Volume Requirements

Why is it essential to collect the correct volume of a blood sample?
Collecting the correct volume ensures enough samples for the laboratory test while preventing excessive blood draw, which can harm the patient. Additionally, incorrect blood-to-additive ratios in collection tubes may lead to erroneous test results.

What might happen if a blood collection tube is underfilled?
Underfilling a tube can lead to an incorrect blood-to-additive ratio, affecting test results' accuracy. For example, underfilling can lead to prolonged clotting times in coagulation tests.

What could occur if a blood collection tube is overfilled?
Overfilling can also result in an incorrect blood-to-additive ratio. Overfilling can lead to a diluted sample and potentially inaccurate test results in tubes with anticoagulants.

How can a phlebotomist ensure they have collected the correct volume?
Most blood collection tubes have a fill line indicating the correct volume. Phlebotomists should fill the tub until this line. For a syringe draw, the book can be read off the syringe.

Can the volume requirements change based on the test to be performed?
Yes, different tests require different volumes of blood. For example, some specialized tests may require larger volumes, while pediatric or capillary collections usually require smaller books. The required text for a specific test should be checked before assembly.

Processing

Chain of Custody Guidelines

What does 'chain of custody' refer to in phlebotomy?
The chain of custody in phlebotomy refers to maintaining control and tracking the handling of a specimen from the moment of collection until the completion of testing. It ensures that the sample has been properly handled and that the test results are associated with the correct patient.

What information is crucial in the chain of custody process?
Essential information includes the patient's identifying details, the date and time of collection, the identity of the collector, and anyone who handled or processed the specimen, including transporters and laboratory technicians.

When is a chain of custody necessary?
Chain of custody is crucial for legal or forensic samples, drug testing, paternity testing, or any tests where results may be used legally. It provides proof that the piece was handled properly and not tampered with.

What could happen if the chain of custody is broken?
The sample's integrity is compromised if the chain of custody is broken or incomplete. This could lead to challenges in court, the invalidation of test results, or the need to recollect the piece.

How can a phlebotomist ensure the chain of custody is maintained?
A phlebotomist can maintain the chain of custody by correctly identifying the patient, appropriately labeling and handling the specimen, recording every person taking the sample, and properly storing it until it reaches the laboratory.

Handling, Storage, and Disposal of Specimens

Why is the correct storage of specimens necessary?
Proper storage of specimens is vital to prevent degradation or changes affecting the test results. Different models require different storage conditions, such as temperature and light exposure.

What are some general guidelines for handling specimens?
General guidelines include handling specimens with clean gloves, avoiding contamination, preventing specimen mix-ups, and delivering samples to the lab as quickly as possible.

How should leftover specimens be disposed of?
Leftover specimens should be disposed of according to the institution's policies and local regulations. They are typically considered biohazardous waste and must be disposed of in designated containers.

What happens if a specimen is not stored at the correct temperature?
Incorrect storage temperatures can lead to changes in the specimen, potentially causing inaccurate test results. For example, some models need refrigeration to slow down metabolic processes, while others must be kept at room temperature.

How can a phlebotomist ensure that they are storing a specimen correctly?
Phlebotomists can refer to laboratory guidelines for storage requirements, including temperature and light conditions. They should also ensure that refrigerators or freezers are functioning correctly.

Centrifugal Techniques

What is the purpose of using a centrifuge in phlebotomy?
A centrifuge is used in phlebotomy to separate the components of a blood sample based on their densities. This allows for the extraction of serum or plasma for various tests.

What factors could affect the outcome of centrifugation?
Factors include the centrifugation speed (revolutions per minute), centrifugation duration, and the sample container type used.

What could happen if a sample needs to be balanced correctly in the centrifuge?
If samples are not balanced, the centrifuge could become unstable during operation, potentially damaging the machine or the examples.

What is the difference between serum and plasma, and how does centrifugation help separate them?
Serum is the liquid portion of the blood after clotting, while plasma is the liquid portion of blood in an anticoagulated sample. Centrifugation separates these components by spinning the blood at high speed, causing the heavier cells to move to the bottom of the tube and leaving the lighter serum or plasma on top.

Why is it essential to avoid hemolysis during centrifugation?
Hemolysis, or the breaking of red blood cells, can release intracellular components that interfere with many tests. Proper handling, including correct centrifugation, can help avoid hemolysis.

Input and Retrieval of Specimen Data in the Information System

Why is it essential to accurately input specimen data into the information system?
Accurate input ensures that test results are associated with the correct patient, test, and sample. It helps avoid errors and misinterpretations.

What information is typically entered into the system when a specimen is collected?
Information typically includes patient identification, specimen type, collection date and time, collector's initials, and any relevant patient information like fasting status or medications.

What are some common errors when entering specimen data into an information system?
Common errors include entering incorrect patient identifiers, selecting the wrong test, incorrect collection date or time, or typos in manual entries.

How can a phlebotomist ensure they are entering data correctly?
Double-checking entries, using barcode scanning when available, and staying familiar with the correct codes and identifiers can help ensure accurate data entry.

Why is it important to know how to retrieve specimen data from the information system?
Retrieving specimen data is necessary for verifying that the correct tests were performed, interpreting results, tracking specimens, and ensuring proper communication of results to healthcare providers.

ADDITIONAL FAQS

Q: What do we mean when talking about Sharp Items?
A: Sharp items comprise needles, syringes, lancets, razor blades, and any object that can penetrate or cut skin. These items must be identified and disposed of properly to avoid injuries and possible passage of infections.

Q: What is the penalty of not disposing of sharps correctly?
A: Healthcare organizations may have to bear fines, other legal issues, and reputational damages arising from penalties associated with improper Sharps disposal. Proper disposal is regulated and essential to ensuring safety and compliance in a healthcare environment.

Q: How would I handle sharp objects that have been discarded carelessly?
A: Avoid managing improperly disposed sharps. Please do not write about it; report the situation to the environment service department of your healthcare facility or the infection control unit. Safe removal and disposal will then be undertaken accordingly.

Q: What measures can healthcare facilities take to avoid wrong sharps disposal?
A: Comprehensive staff training availability of properly labeled sharps containers for every healthcare facility, with strict regular auditing and maintaining of the cultural norm, should be undertaken by healthcare facilities to eliminate improper sharps disposal. Preventing inappropriate removals involves education and awareness.

Q: Are sharps disposal containers reusable?
A: Never should sharps disposal containers be reused! These single-use containers are put in place to preserve the integrity of the waste containment system and eliminate any contaminations. Containers should be used just once since reusing them erodes their usefulness and can endanger healthcare workers and the environment.

Q: How should you document Patient Consent in Phlebotomy?
A: In phlebotomy, the best way to do this is by having a particular consent form, which states the reasons for taking blood, the risk attached, and possible alternatives. Then, a patient or the concerned legal representative shall sign and date the form as an affirmation of acceptance.

Q: Does a phlebotomy offer an opportunity for withdrawal of consent for a patient?
A: At any time, a patient can choose to opt out of the process of phlebotomy. Phlebotomists should listen to what the patient says verbally or nonverbally and immediately stop the procedure if they withdraw consent to continue.

Q: What should phlebotomists do to ensure they have received informed consent?
A: The phlebotomist should explain the procedure fully, answer patients' questions if necessary, and confirm that the patient understands and agrees. Appropriate consent forms must be in writing, and understanding verification must be recorded verbally.

Q: What if a patient cannot provide consent?
A: Following established protocols and regulations, the phlebotomist should seek consent from a legally authorized representative of the patient if they cannot support themselves due to mental impairment or other reasons.

Q: What do phlebotomists do on needles' phobias?
A: Needle phobia in phlebotomists can be addressed through recognizing the patients' fears, offering comfort, and using distraction methods. Open communication, a comfortable environment, and tiny gauge needles may also quell worry.

Q: What specific considerations should be made for this group of patients?
A: In phlebotomy, special considerations for geriatric patients are ascertaining frailty, providing comfort, and allowing enough procedure time. To provide good care, optimal clear communication, gentle handling, and close attention to the possible coexistence of other diseases must be observed.

Q: What is your policy on collecting blood from a post-mastectomy patient?
A: Taking blood from such a patient should be done by using the contralateral arm or applying distal veins on the same side. Sensitivity to the patient's physical and mental welfare, getting informed consent, and adjusting techniques are essential.

Q: If a patient suffers from a blood disorder such as hemophilia, what action needs to be taken?
A: Phlebotomy entails close coordination with the patient's healthcare team as they deal with the patient with a blood disorder like hemophilia. It includes selection of proper venipuncture sites and additional precautionary measures to minimize bleeding. Informed consent and close patient observation before, during, and post-procedure are crucial.

Q: What would help to calm a child down for a blood test?
A: A pediatric patient is comfortable sticking his arm for the blood-letting exercise in a manner explained using age-appropriate language and involving some distractions such as toys and games. Guiding calmly and reassuringly promotes trust between the teacher and the child's family.

Q: What are the best approaches to overcome an obstinate venipuncture in an obese patient?
A: When confronted with such tough cases of difficult venipuncture caused by obesity, it is essential to use proper gear. Palpation should be used to identify the accessible venous points, and one needs alternative venipuncture spots. Establishing clear communication with the patient and adjusting techniques to suit the patient's physical needs should be considered when performing a successful blood draw.

Q: Is there any way to calm a nervous patient before a blood draw?
A: Calming a nervous patient before performing a blood draw can involve giving detailed explanations, incorporating relaxation methods, providing alternative distractions, and creating a favorable atmosphere. Furthermore, empathy and actively hearing out the patient's worries will also quell this anxiety.

Q: How do you handle a situation where a patient has waited for very long hours only to get delayed as far as the procedure is concerned?
A: Apologizing for the inconvenience and offering a short but apparent reason for the postponement is very important in this case. In addition, one must ensure the patient that their time matters. It is worth noting that offering options for rescheduling and prioritization of urgent issues helps manage patient expectations.

Q: What is the appropriate action for a phlebotomist if a patient gets angry or upset when undergoing a blood draw?
A: If a patient experiences anger or frustration, phlebotomists must keep calm, acknowledge those experiences, and respond kindly. If it becomes inevitable, suspend the process, grant the patient time to allow them to unburden themselves emotionally, and recommend that the process start again once they are willing to cooperate.

Q: How can phlebotomists show respect for their patients' privacy to ensure the confidentiality of their personal information?

A: Privacy and confidentiality require that phlebotomists provide a private and safe place for drawing blood into some quiet environment. Discreet communication and handling of patient information as required by legal instruments such as HIPAA are also needed here.

Q: Why does body language matter in patient communication?
A: The professionalism of medical personnel concerning body language employed while interacting with their patients is highly pivotal in demonstrating empathy and reassurance. Having an open, upright position with frequent looks at patients while maintaining concentration on their nonverbal messages enhances a friendly atmosphere for the client.

Q: What should be some of these approaches for phlebotomists toward culturally sensitive patient' preparation?
A: To have a culture-sensitive approach, phlebotomists must be aware of various cultural practices, ask open-ended questions to ascertain personalized options, and respect people's beliefs. Patient-centeredness involves adapting one's communication style and awareness of culture.

Q: What should phlebotomists consider when conducting a blood draw upon a disabled patient or client?
A: Phlebotomists should also ask questions about special requirements for disabled patients; they will need to give help or make the service procedures suitable for patients. This could entail the provision of wheelchair areas, adjustment of bed height, or working together with support staff to guarantee a hitch-free stay.

Q: What strategies do phlebotomists use to overcome language barriers in their patients who are not English speakers?
A: It also entails engaging with professional interpreters' services, using different multilingual information materials, and employing visual aids to facilitate understanding. Ensuring patient readiness involves explaining clearly how a venesection is done and obtaining consent using their preferred language.

Q: What considerations should be made when preparing pediatric patients for blood collection?
A: There are several ways of considering preparations that can be done for pediatric patients. These considerations include using age-appropriate communication methods, making the environment child-friendly, and allowing the presence of parents or guardians should they wish to be in the procedure room. Gentle approaches and distraction techniques will help phlebotomists create good experiences for the child.

Q: What adjustments do phlebotomists make in dealing with patients who have been traumatized before?
A: Phlebotomists should, therefore, be sensitive while conducting any procedures on patients who have previously experienced trauma. The phlebotomy technician should also ask if there are any particular areas they want to avoid or anything else that may provoke their memories of pain and discomfort as they try to communicate. In such cases, creating trust and ensuring good communication is crucial.

Q: On taking blood, what measures may phlebotomists adopt to minimize pain and discomfort?
A: Phlebotomists should use appropriate-sized needles for painless blood collection; a warm compress can also be applied, but distraction is essential. A more amiable experience is fostered by communicating with the patient, curbing anxieties, and working effectively.

Q: What are the guidelines for addressing the issue of blood clotting in the patients undergoing treatment of which phlebotomists could potentially be affected?
A: Phlebotomists should seek information on medicines involved in clot disruption, where appropriate, take additional care during venipuncture, and cooperate with other health professionals. The necessary consideration is adopting techniques to treat the area with pain and the site of the wound through which the individual may have lost a lot of blood.

Q: What are the difficulties of collecting blood samples from dehydrated patients?
A: Taking blood samples from a patient can pose a challenge in cases of dehydration, where blood volume is significantly low, and there may not be enough vascularity. Therefore, phlebotomists must ensure proper hydration for the sample given, explore other potential venipuncture alternatives, and inform the patient of possible difficulties that can be expected to manage expectations correctly.

Q: What can phlebotomists do about patient anxiousness due to the blood extraction procedure?
A: Since this may cause patient anxiety, it is essential to be honest with them about what will happen, why they are doing the test, as well as any worries that the client may have. Besides distractions and practicing empathy, a calm and relaxing setting should also be developed, which helps reduce anxiety and improves the patient's experience.

Q: What is the leading equipment for everyday venipuncture?
A: The everyday things used in normal venipuncture include tourniquets, alcohol swabs or antibacterial wipes; adhesive bands, needle holders or winged injectable syringes; blood collection tubes/ syringes; and biohazardous waste receipt

Q: Why should an individual assemble all other items before proceeding with a venipuncture process?
A: Pre-assembling all necessary equipment, including disposable syringes, alcohol swabs, and gauzes, before initiating venipuncture ensures that it is done with care and without exposing health workers or patients to infections. This allows phlebotomists to focus on the process and the patient without any disruption/delay.

Q: What factors must be considered when selecting the right venipuncture needle?
A: Factors to consider when picking up an appropriate needle for venipuncture are related to the patient's vein size and condition, the kind of blood collection system, and the use of the blood draw. Choosing the correct gauge and length makes the whole process smooth and pleasant for the patient and the doctor.

Q: When does it become expedient to resort to a butterfly needle in phlebotomy?
A: In cases where a butterfly needle is used during phlebotomy in small and fragile veins, like in pediatric or old patients, it would be beneficial to have in-depth knowledge about the process. It offers more precision and reduces the stress on the brittle vein system.

Q: How can the safety and cleanliness of phlebotomy equipment be achieved?
A: Inspect worn or damaged equipment for safety; observe sterilization and disinfection procedures; and abide by infection control protocol. The other measure involves using single-use and disposable items as often as possible to minimize contamination chances.

Q: What does the order of draw mean in phlebotomy?
A: Phlebotomy relies on draw order to prevent contamination between blood collection tubes, thus leading to accurate testing and avoidance of any errors. This ensures that the proper sequence is followed so as not to have any additive from one line contaminating the other tubes, preserving separate specimens.

Q: How should venipuncture be taken?
A: In venipuncture, the preferred draw of the order is blood culture bottles, coagulate bottles, serous bottles, heparin bottles, eta, and tubes from different additives. The latter sequence is considered safe as it reduces tube cross-contamination.

Q: What are the main objectives of OSHA regulations as applied to healthcare?
A: OSHA regulations in health care focus on protecting both staff and patients through regulation of workplace safety, including handling of hazardous materials, infection control, and use of suitable protective gear.

Q: What is the role of HIPAA in protecting patients?
A: Under HIPAA, PHI is regulated by a series of guidelines governing its access, use, and disclosure. It involves ensuring that security procedures like encryption, secure transmission, and patient consent are complied with by healthcare providers whenever they seek to share their knowledge.

Q: Describe some widely used quality control steps in phlebotomy.
A: Proper patient identification procedures, strict technical specimen collection, implementation of standard operating procedures, frequent instrument calibration procedures, and continuous proficiency testing programs are necessary standard quality control measures in phlebotomy. Taken together, these measures guarantee the authenticity and the credibility of laboratory findings.

Q: Why does poor quality control matter in health care?
A: Quality control in healthcare involves providing accurate test results, correct diagnoses, effective treatment procedures, safe patients, and improved healthcare system reliability. This may also put healthcare organizations under legal and financial sanction.

Q: What measures should healthcare professionals employ for quality assurance?
A: Through this, professionals in healthcare can ascertain that best practices are maintained, participate in continuing education, observe proper protocols, engage in frequent self-assessment, and promote a sense of responsibility among workmates. Regular audits and quality improvement programs are also necessary.

Q: What part can continuous improvement play in quality control?
A: Quality control entails a continuous improvement process that includes assessing and revising healthcare practices about efficiency, precision, and patient success. Through this process, healthcare organizations identify ways to improve themselves to meet emerging standards of quality care delivery.

Q: How should healthcare discard sharps?
A: After using used needles and other sharp objects, they must be placed into puncture-resistant containers to handle sharps in healthcare settings properly. They are subsequently placed in containers and locked up safely before disposal by local biosafety laws.

Q: What is the significance of proper sharps disposal?
A: Sharp disposal must be done correctly to avert accidental puncture wound injuries, lower the risk of infecting others, and shield healthcare workers and members of the public from danger. It's essential for infection control, contributing to workplace safety.

Q: In case healthcare workers experience needle stick injuries, what is their following action?
A: On being pricked by a used needle, healthcare workers should first wash the site with soap and water, then report the event to their superior and seek immediate medical care. Early intervention reduces the risk of transmitting an infection or related health issues.

Q: How can I deal with a case where the sharps disposal container is full?
A: If the sharps container is full, healthcare personnel must follow established procedures for closing and sealing such a container, replacing it with another new one, and ensuring all required labels are in place. Disposing promptly of full containers is essential to keep the surroundings safe and healthy.

Q: Is it okay to throw sharps into the common trash?
A: Should sharps not be put into the conventional trashing? Disposal must be done in proper containers, called the sharps container, to prevent accidents and conform to OSHA biohazards standards. Throwing sharps in regular trash is a hazardous way to dispose of them, as it creates various safety and environmental issues.

Q: Are there any commonly accepted practices used in healthcare organizations today?
A: Standard practices in the healthcare setting encompass guidelines on patient treatment, hygiene regulations, documentation, employee education, and a clean, secure environment. They set up standards that ensure the smooth running of the health facilities.

Q: What do ethics entail in health care, and why is it important?
A: Ethics in healthcare helps professionals make righteous decisions. They develop patient trust, enhance transparency, and uphold ethics in health care. Issues like patient confidentiality and consent of the patients and equitable access to care are included in the ethical standards.

Q: What is the cost of violating OSHA's regulations?
A: The healthcare setting imposes high fines and even legal consequences for failing to adhere to OSHA directives. Such sentences may differ depending on the type of violation and its seriousness, underlining the necessity to prevent threatening health staff and patients' lives.

Q: What does HIPAA define as PHI?
A: According to HIPAA, PHI includes any health data that concerns an individual's physical or mental wellness, which can serve as identifying information associated with them in any manner concerning their past, present, or future physical, mental, and payment condition. This includes but is not limited to extensive sets like medical records and insurance bills.

Q: What measures should caregivers take to guarantee operation compliance?
A: To achieve compliance with operational standards, healthcare professionals may keep themselves updated on guidelines, attend training courses, and implement appropriate procedures. Continuous audits, self-assessment, and team communication also help keep the highest operating standards.

Q: Give one example of an ethical dilemma in healthcare.
A: Ethical challenges that arise in the context of health care may be related to revealing an imminent death to a patient when the families disagree with such disclosure. Healthcare providers face an ethical dilemma that requires balancing honesty, patient autonomy, and family issues.

Q: What is OSHA's method of ensuring safety in the workplace?
A: OSHA conducts routine inspections, investigates complaints, and inflicts financial punishments upon companies failing to comply with standards. Further, they offer educational guides and materials that enable healthcare entities to understand better and execute the safety protocols.

Q: What measures should healthcare organizations implement to achieve HIPAA compliance?
A: Compliance of healthcare organizations with HIPAA can be ensured through a comprehensive training program, enforcing access controls, periodic risk assessment, and updating privacy policies periodically. These measures are preventive approaches guaranteeing the confidentiality of patients' information and adherence to the law.

Q: What makes quality control an essential part of healthcare?
A: Healthcare quality control must be ensured for accurate diagnosis and treatment of patients and overall quality service provision. It reduces errors, increases the security of patients, and contributes to trust in the healthcare system through the achievement of good practices.

Q: What do phlebotomists do about quality control?
A: Phlebotomists' participation in quality control is about specifying, accurately managing, and precisely taking blood specimens for analysis. These professionals use standard protocols for reliable testing outcomes to reduce all possible pre-analytical errors from the laboratory tests, leading to accurate diagnosis and good patient management.

Q: Give an instance of a quality control method used for a medical practice.
A: Quality control in a health care facility could entail recalibration of medical equipment like blood pressure monitors and laboratory instruments for accuracy each time. By being proactive, it is possible to discover and correct any departures from set standards concerning patient care quality.

Q: What impact does quality control have on patient service?
A: Quality control ensures minimal errors in patients' diagnoses and treatment. This improves the accuracy of medical test results, provides standardization within healthcare activities, and yields better patient experiences and outcomes, among other things.

Q: What are the keys to remembering the order we draw?
A: With some standard mnemonics, one may remember the draw order, "Stoplight; green light, go." Blood culture tube, coagulation tube, heparin (separation) tube, gel separator tube, and "others" such as EDTA.

Q: Why should the draw order be followed in this process?
A: Improper following of order of draw increases the threat of specimen contamination. Transferring additives from one tube will likely lead to false results, compromising patients' diagnosis and treatment.

Q: Do drawing orders vary using a syringe or the evacuated tube system?
A: However, syringe versus evacuated tube systems may have different draw orders. The charge is based on the tube's additive requirements when used with a needle or designed to prevent cross-contamination in an evacuated tube system.

Q: Can one palpate the venipuncture site after applying the antiseptic agent?
A: Yes, one is allowed to palpate at the venipuncture site to locate a vein following the use of an antiseptic agent. To perform an appropriate blood draw, palpation locates suitable and usable veins. Palpation of the site should only be done after ensuring that the antiseptic dries up first so as not to contaminate.

Q: Why should an antiseptic be used during finger stick and heel stick procedures?
A: It is essential to use antiseptic agents for procedures involving finger sticks or heel sticks to prevent infections. Although these approaches are non-invasive compared to venipuncture, maintaining an aseptic process remains paramount for the patient's security.

Q: How should you fill in a specimen label?
A: The specimen label shall contain the patient's full name, date of birth, a unique identification number, date and time of collection, the phlebotomist's initials, and whatever else may be required by individual laboratories or facilities' protocols.

Q: When should specimens be labeled?
A: Upon collecting specimens, the patient's presence should be used to label the samples immediately. Every employee within a company should have a clearly defined task or role based on their specific responsibilities and functions within the organization. This facilitates correct and identifiable specification tagging, thus minimizing the chances of wrong labeling and enhancing the reliability of tests.

Q: What would be the possible effects of poor labeling on a specimen?
A: An example here is improper labeling on a specimen that can result in misidentification with wrongful tests and, therefore, cause patient damage. Labeling should be put in place to ensure the specimen's integrity and correct diagnosis and possible treatment.

Q: How should care be administered post-procedure after a venipuncture?
A: The post-procedure care of a venipuncture involves placing a sterile dressing on the puncture point, achieving good hemostasis, giving due instructions to the patients, and observing unfavorable reactions that might occur. Additionally, the process and the patient's response must be documented.

Q: How long should one continue applying pressure to a venipuncture site after removing the needle?
A: One should press a venipuncture site for about one minute or two until there is no more blood flow from that point. This minimizes hematoma formation as well as assists in proper clotting.

Q: What should I recommend to an ex-patient after the venipuncture procedure?
A: The patients are advised to keep the bandage on for a few hours, abstain from performing heavy labor using the arm or engaging in some strenuous activities for some time, and report any abnormal symptoms or complications that include excess bleeding, swelling, infection, etc.

Q: Which symptoms of an infection after a procedure should I be aware of?
A: Patients are advised to look out for these after-procedure indicators of postoperative infection: redness, swellings, warmth, and drainage/discharging. Healthcare providers should also promptly report other symptoms, such as fever, chills, and persistent pain, for further investigation.

Q: What kind of non-blood specimens can a phlebotomist be asked to draw from?
A: A phlebotomist may also be required to collect non-blood specimens, including, for example, urine, stool, sputum, saliva, cerebrospinal fluid, and other body fluids or tissue for laboratory diagnostic testing.

Q: How should a urine specimen be collected?
A: The required approach in obtaining a urine sample is the midstream, clean catch procedure. The patient is made to excrete just a little urine, discard the primary stream, and save some mid-stream urine in a sterile container.

Q: When collecting a stool sample, what information should a doctor give a patient?
A: Patients should be advised to collect a stool sample in a clean bottle without any toilet water or cleaning agents. Some special instructions may involve not taking some laxatives and certain medications that can affect the test results.

Q: What makes it necessary to label a non-blood specimen correctly?
A: Proper labeling is imperative to get an effective and correct identification and record keeping of a non-blood specimen. Correct tagging is necessary to correctly associate the sample with a particular patient, ultimately reducing wrong diagnoses or treatments.

Q: How do you handle non-blood specimen samples?
A: Nonblood specimens must be handled with care, observing specimen integrity, proper storage conditions (refrigeration where necessary), and the facility's protocols regarding transporting samples and processing.

Q: Why does a venipuncture require prior skin preparation?
A: A venipuncture preceded by skin preparation helps minimize infection risk. It removes surface bacteria to ensure an aseptic environment suitable for injection and an uncontaminated sample of drawn blood.

Q: What reagent do you mainly use for prepping a patient's skin when performing routine venipunctures?
A: Isopropyl alcohol remains the most common agent for skin preparation during routine venipuncture. This helps minimize levels of microbes on the skin, promoting aseptic measures for the venipuncture technique.

Q: How do I apply the antiseptic agent on the skin?
A: The back-to-back pattern in applying the agent is correct at the skin's center and towards the periphery. The method eliminates bacteria in and around the wound surface, thus clearing the path of bacteria without forcing them more deeply within the hole.

Q: Is it possible to touch the injection area once an antiseptic is applied?
A: Once applied, the antiseptic should never touch the venipuncture site. Bacteria may come from any contact, destroying the sterilization and raising the risk of infections.

Q: What should you do if a patient is allergic to the antiseptic agent?
A: Alternative antiseptic is recommended for patients allergic to antiseptic agents after ensuring the patient's history of allergy. We are identifying a proper and secure substitute through communication with the patient and cooperation with healthcare providers.

Q: What makes it essential for the proper blood specimen volume?
A: Blood collection should be done precisely to obtain an adequate quantity for testing. This can result in sample rejection or correct readings, impacting the patients' diagnosis and management regimen.

Q: What happens if a blood collection tube is overfilling?
A: Excess blood into the blood collection tube could change the blood/additive ratio, causing wrong test results. Filling lines beyond capacity creates problems during centrifugation, causing hemolysis and sample rejection.

Q: What steps can a phlebotomist take to confirm they have drawn an adequate amount?
A: To ensure the correct volume has been collected, phlebotomists should follow tube fill protocols, use suitable collection tubes, and observe the volume marks drawn on evacuated tubes. Accurate specimen collection is a result of proper training as well as following the set procedures.

Q: Can the volume requirements be varied depending on the specific test?
A: However, these quantities could vary depending on a specific test in specific. The amount of blood required for lab tests varies depending on the type of test performed. Therefore, phlebotomists must know the exact volume needed for every test.

Q: Why is there necessarily a need for fasting in some tests done on blood samples?
A: Certain blood tests require fasting to provide baseline measures that are as accurate and true as possible. It is easier to measure an individual's current metabolism as fasting helps cleanse any recent effects of food intake, such as elevating or disturbing the results of blood sugar, lipid concentration, etc.

Q: Guidelines for instructing a patient for 24 hours of urine.
A: The patient should be asked to discard the first-morning void, collect all other urine in 24 hours, keep the container refrigerated during the procedure, and note any missed collections.

Q: What should the phlebotomist do if the collected sample is grossly contaminated?
A: A phlebotomist should also not collect or process the sample if it demonstrates contamination. Instead, they alert the healthcare team, document the issue, and recall the selection using the correct procedures.

PRACTICE TEST

A part from academic assistance, here are 120 Multiple Choice Questions classified into all five parts of the NHA Phlebotomy exam syllabus. These can help you to assess yourself and prepare better for the exam!

Safety and Compliance

1. What does OSHA primarily regulate in the field of phlebotomy?
   - **A.** Patient billing
   - **B.** Employee safety
   - **C.** Medical records management
   - **D.** Clinical trial protocols

2. Which act safeguards patient privacy and confidentiality in the healthcare setting?
   - **A.** OSHA
   - **B.** HIPAA
   - **C.** CLIA
   - **D.** FDA

3. Which of the following is not considered a biohazardous sharp?
   - **A.** Scalpel
   - **B.** Lancet
   - **C.** Suture needle
   - **D.** Blood pressure cuff

4. Which item is not a type of PPE?
   - **A.** Gloves
   - **B.** Lab coat
   - **C.** Goggles
   - **D.** Stethoscope

5. What is the recommended minimum time for effective handwashing?
   - **A.** 5 seconds
   - **B.** 10 seconds
   - **C.** 20 seconds
   - **D.** 1 minute

6. What should be done if a phlebotomist is exposed to a patient's blood through a needlestick injury?
   - **A.** Ignore it if the patient is known to be healthy.
   - **B.** Wash the area with soap and water, then report the incident.
   - **C.** Apply a bandage and continue working.
   - **D.** Rinse the area with bleach.

7. What is the purpose of quality control in a laboratory setting?
   - **A.** To ensure accurate and reliable test results.
   - **B.** To decrease costs.
   - **C.** To increase test volume.
   - **D.** To minimize personnel needs.

8. In which container should contaminated needles be disposed of?
   A. Regular trash can
   B. Recycling bin
   C. Sharps container
   D. Biohazard waste bag

9. What is the first thing a phlebotomist should do after removing gloves?
   A. Document the procedure
   B. Dispose of the gloves in the regular trash
   C. Wash hands
   D. Put on a new pair of gloves

10. What is the primary purpose of infection control in phlebotomy?
    A. Protecting patients from infections that can be transmitted by blood
    B. Protecting the phlebotomist from bloodborne pathogens
    C. Both A and B
    D. Neither A nor B

11. What is the main reason for ethical standards in the healthcare setting?
    A. To promote high standards of practice.
    B. To attract more patients to the facility.
    C. To ensure that all staff members get along.
    D. To ensure a higher salary for employees.

12. Which of the following should a phlebotomist do to adhere to HIPAA regulations?
    A. Discuss patient information in the break room.
    B. Leave patient results visible on a computer screen.
    C. Share patient records with friends who work in healthcare.
    D. Store patient information securely and disclose it only to authorized personnel.

13. Which of the following does NOT represent a phlebotomist's adherence to OSHA guidelines?
    A. Disposing of sharps in a designated sharps container.
    B. Wearing PPE when handling blood and bodily fluids.
    C. Eating and drinking in the phlebotomy lab.
    D. Following procedures to prevent needlestick injuries.

14. How should a phlebotomist manage a contaminated sharp?
    A. Throw it in the regular waste bin.
    B. Wash it off and reuse it.
    C. Dispose of it in a designated sharps container.
    D. Leave it on the phlebotomy tray for cleaning later.

15. What should be done if a chemical spill occurs in the lab?
    A. Ignore it if it is small.
    B. Leave it for the janitorial staff to clean.
    C. Wash it down the drain with water.
    D. Follow the facility's spill cleanup procedures.

16. What is the first step to take when an exposure incident occurs?
    A. Continue working and report the incident later.
    B. Clean the exposed area and report the incident.
    C. Go home and seek medical attention later.
    D. Ignore the incident if the exposed individual does not feel sick.

17. What is the most critical component of hand hygiene?
  A. Using hot water
  B. Using antibacterial soap
  C. Washing for at least 20 seconds
  D. Drying hands on a clean towel

18. When is it acceptable to not wear PPE?
  A. When the patient is a known relative
  B. When the phlebotomist is not in a patient room
  C. When the procedure does not involve blood or body fluids
  D. It is always necessary to wear PPE.

19. What is quality control in phlebotomy mainly concerned with?
  A. Ensuring the phlebotomist does not work overtime
  B. Ensuring that specimens are collected, stored, and handled correctly
  C. Making sure the phlebotomist takes their lunch break
  D. Making sure all patients are happy with their care

20. What does the term "exposure control" mean in a healthcare setting?
  A. Controlling patient exposure to the sun
  B. Controlling access to patient records
  C. Controlling the exposure of healthcare workers to potentially infectious materials
  D. Controlling patient exposure to cold temperatures

Patient Preparation

1. Which of the following is the most effective way for a phlebotomist to establish rapport with a patient?
   A. Talk about personal life.
   B. Ask the patient about their personal life.
   C. Use clear, understandable language and show empathy.
   D. Avoid unnecessary conversation.

2. What is the first step before obtaining a blood sample from a patient?
   A. Prepare the equipment.
   B. Obtain informed consent.
   C. Apply the tourniquet.
   D. Clean the puncture site.

3. A patient has a fear of needles. What should the phlebotomist consider this?
   A. A reason to refuse service.
   B. An annoyance.
   C. A special consideration.
   D. Irrelevant to the procedure.

4. What should a phlebotomist consider when choosing a vein for venipuncture?
   A. The patient's preference.
   B. The size, condition, and location of the vein.
   C. The phlebotomist's preference.
   D. The color of the vein.

5. What instructions might a phlebotomist give to a patient providing a urine specimen?
   A. "Ensure to fill the cup."
   B. "Start urinating in the toilet, then collect mid-stream."
   C. "Collect the sample in your home toilet and bring it to the lab."
   D. "Drink plenty of water right before collecting the sample."

6. Why is timing crucial in specific blood tests?
   A. It affects the phlebotomist's schedule.
   B. It can impact the accuracy of the test results.
   C. It impacts the patient's comfort during the procedure.
   D. It affects the billing of the procedure.

7. When should a patient be informed about the purpose of a blood draw?
   A. After the procedure.
   B. During the procedure.
   C. Just before the procedure.
   D. At the time of scheduling the procedure.

8. A patient has a history of syncope during blood draws. What is this considered during the pre-draw assessment?
   A. An inconvenience.
   B. A contraindication for the procedure.
   C. A special consideration.
   D. A reason to refer the patient to a physician.

9. Why should a phlebotomist avoid drawing blood from the arm on the same side as a mastectomy?
   A. The veins in that arm are likely damaged.
   B. The patient may experience discomfort.
   C. It's against the law.
   D. It can increase the risk of lymphedema.

10. Which patients might require special instructions when giving a stool sample?
    A. A patient who has never been given a stool sample before.
    B. A patient who has given stool samples before.
    C. A patient who has a urinary tract infection.
    D. A patient who has diarrhea.

11. When should a phlebotomist communicate the procedure's purpose to the patient?
    A. Just before the procedure.
    B. After the procedure.
    C. During the procedure.
    D. As soon as the patient arrives at the lab.

12. What is the appropriate response when a patient declines a blood draw?
    A. Proceed with the blood draw anyway.
    B. Inform the patient that they have no choice.
    C. Respect the patient's decision and notify the appropriate healthcare provider.
    D. Try to convince the patient that it's not painful.

13. How can a phlebotomist assist a patient with needle phobia?
    A. By drawing blood as quickly as possible.
    B. By minimizing discussion about the needle.
    C. By showing the patient the needle beforehand.
    D. By applying a topical anesthetic and providing reassurance.

14. What's the recommended site for capillary blood collection in adults?
    A. The heel.
    B. The fingertip.
    C. The forearm.
    D. The antecubital area.

15. How long should a tourniquet be left on during a venipuncture?
    A. Less than 1 minute.
    B. 2 to 3 minutes.
    C. As long as it takes to draw blood.
    D. Until the vein is visible.

16. What should the phlebotomist do if a patient becomes dizzy during a blood draw?
    A. Continue with the draw and finish quickly.
    B. Ask the patient to breathe deeply and slowly.
    C. Tell the patient it will pass and try to relax.
    D. Leave the patient alone to recover.

17. What is important to remember when drawing a glucose tolerance test (GTT)?
    A. The patient must be fasting.
    B. The draw must occur in the morning.
    C. The patient must be hydrated.
    D. The draw must occur after the patient exercises.

What should a phlebotomist do if a patient faints during a venipuncture procedure?
- **A.** Complete the venipuncture as quickly as possible.
- **B.** Leave the patient and seek help.
- **C.** Immediately remove the needle and lower the patient's head.
- **D.** Ask the patient to stand up and walk around.

18. What is the most appropriate location for an infant heel stick?
- **A.** The center of the heel.
- **B.** The side of the heel.
- **C.** The top of the foot.
- **D.** The toe.

19. What is the primary reason for patient identification during phlebotomy?
- **A.** To bill the patient for services rendered.
- **B.** To ensure the correct patient is being tested.
- **C.** To comply with healthcare privacy laws.
- **D.** To create a patient profile in the laboratory information system.

20. What type of specimen is typically collected for a urine pregnancy test?
- **A.** First-morning urine.
- **B.** Random urine.
- **C.** 24-hour urine.
- **D.** Midstream clean-catch urine.

21. What is essential to consider when drawing blood from a geriatric patient?
- **A.** Draw from the same vein every time.
- **B.** Use a larger needle to ensure a good flow.
- **C.** Use a tourniquet as tight as possible.
- **D.** Veins may be more fragile and prone to bruising.

22. When should a phlebotomist wash their hands?
- **A.** Before and after each patient contact.
- **B.** Only after contact with blood or body fluids.
- **C.** Only at the beginning and end of the shift.
- **D.** Only if the phlebotomist feels their hands are dirty.

23. How should a phlebotomist respond if a patient refuses to have blood drawn?
- **A.** Insist that the test is essential and continue with the procedure.
- **B.** Respect the patient's decision, inform the patient's healthcare provider, and document the incident.
- **C.** Call the patient's family and ask them to convince the patient.
- **D.** Tell the patient that refusal may result in a delay in diagnosis or treatment.

24. How can a phlebotomist prevent needlestick injuries?
- **A.** By recapping needles after use.
- **B.** By using a safety-engineered needle and following proper disposal procedures.
- **C.** By throwing used needles directly into the trash can.
- **D.** By washing hands before and after each patient contact.

Routine Blood Collections

1. Which piece of equipment should be prepared first for a blood draw?
   A. Tourniquet
   B. Alcohol wipes
   C. Needle and holder
   D. Test tubes

2. When doing a multi-tube draw, what is the correct order of interest?
   A. Green, lavender, red, gray
   B. Red, green, lavender, gray
   C. Blue, red, green, lavender
   D. Blue, red, lavender, green

3. Which antiseptic agent is commonly used in a routine venipuncture?
   A. Iodine
   B. Chlorhexidine
   C. Hydrogen peroxide
   D. Isopropyl alcohol

4. What information must be included when labeling a specimen?
   A. patient's full name, date of birth, date and time of collection, and phlebotomist's initials
   B. Patient's full name, date and time of collection, and phlebotomist's initials
   C. Patient's full name, age, and date of collection
   D. Patient's full name, date of birth, and date of collection

5. After removing the needle from the patient's arm, what is the first step in post-procedure care?
   A. Discard the needle in a sharps container.
   B. Apply pressure to the venipuncture site.
   C. Label the collection tubes.
   D. Thank the patient.

6. After completing the blood draw, when should the phlebotomist remove their gloves?
   A. Immediately after removing the needle from the patient's arm.
   B. After applying pressure and a bandage to the venipuncture site.
   C. After labeling the blood collection tubes.
   D. After disposing of the used needle and holder in a sharps container.

7. Why is it important to follow the correct draw order when collecting multiple samples from a single venipuncture?
   A. To ensure patient comfort.
   B. To prevent cross-contamination of additives between tubes.
   C. To make sure all tubes are filled.
   D. To minimize the time the tourniquet is applied.

8. What is the correct angle for needle insertion during venipuncture?
   A. 15-30 degrees.
   B. 35-45 degrees.
   C. 50-60 degrees.
   D. 70-80 degrees.

9. When should you release the tourniquet during the venipuncture procedure?
   A. Before inserting the needle.
   B. Immediately after inserting the needle.
   C. After blood starts to flow into the tube.
   D. After removing the needle from the arm.

10. Why is it essential to invert the tubes after collecting a blood sample?
    A. To mix the blood with the additives in the tube.
    B. To prevent clotting.
    C. To ensure a full draw.
    D. To prevent hemolysis.

11. How should sharps be disposed of after a blood draw?
    A. In a regular trash can
    B. In a biohazard bag
    C. In a sharps container
    D. In a recycling bin

12. What is the purpose of wearing Personal Protective Equipment (PPE) during a venipuncture procedure?
    A. To protect the phlebotomist from exposure to blood and other body fluids
    B. To make the patient feel more comfortable
    C. To ensure a successful blood draw
    D. To follow hospital policy

13. What is the first step to take after a needlestick injury?
    A. Report the incident to a supervisor
    B. Immediately wash the area with soap and water
    C. Apply a bandage to the area
    D. Continue with the blood draw procedure

14. Why must the lid be placed on a specimen tube after collection?
    A. To prevent spillage
    B. To prevent evaporation
    C. To prevent exposure to air
    D. All of the above

15. Why should the patient's arm be positioned downward during venipuncture?
    A. To prevent the patient from seeing the procedure
    B. To facilitate blood flow
    C. To minimize discomfort
    D. To stabilize the arm

16. Which response is most appropriate if a patient faints during a venipuncture procedure?
    A. Continue with the procedure and alert a supervisor afterward.
    B. Immediately remove the needle, apply pressure to the site, and position the patient in a way to restore blood flow to the brain.
    C. Call for help while continuing to draw blood.
    D. Immediately remove the needle and finish the draw from the other arm.

17. If a patient has a mastectomy on the left side, which arm should be used for the blood draw?
    A. The left arm
    B. The right arm
    C. Either arm, it doesn't matter
    D. Neither arm, a leg should be used instead

18. Which is best to mix a blood sample with an anticoagulant in a collection tube?
    A. Shaking the tube vigorously
    B. Stirring with a small rod
    C. Inverting the tube gently several times
    D. Rotating the tube end-to-end

19. What is the correct draw order for a complete blood count (CBC), coagulation test (PT/INR), and electrolyte panel?
    A. Coagulation tube, CBC tube, electrolyte panel tube
    B. CBC tube, electrolyte panel tube, coagulation tube
    C. Electrolyte panel tube, CBC tube, coagulation tube
    D. Coagulation tube, electrolyte panel tube, CBC tube

20. What should you do if you cannot find a suitable vein for venipuncture after applying a tourniquet?
    A. Try to draw blood from a vein that is not visible but can be palpated.
    B. Have the patient dangle their arm to increase blood flow and try again.
    C. Apply a warm compress to the area to make the veins more visible.
    D. All of the above.

21. Which antiseptic agent is most commonly used for routine venipuncture?
    A. Povidone-iodine
    B. Chlorhexidine
    C. Hydrogen peroxide
    D. Isopropyl alcohol

22. Which of the following statements about patient identification is correct?
    A. It's okay to draw blood if the patient's ID band is missing as long as they verbally confirm their identity.
    B. The phlebotomist should compare the information on the requisition form to the patient's ID band.
    C. The patient's bed number is sufficient for identification purposes.
    D. The phlebotomist should identify the patient by their full name and date of birth.

23. When performing a venipuncture, the needle's bevel should face the following:
    A. Downward
    B. Upward
    C. Sideways
    D. The direction doesn't matter

24. You are about to draw blood, and the patient suddenly withdraws their arm and refuses the procedure. What should you do?
    A. Proceed with the draw, as the tests are medically necessary.
    B. Try to convince the patient by telling them the procedure won't hurt.
    C. Stop the procedure, inform the patient's healthcare provider, and document the incident.
    D. Tell the patient they have no choice but to have the procedure.

25. What is the first thing you should do after successfully performing venipuncture and filling the tubes?
    A. Remove the tourniquet.
    B. Apply a bandage to the site.
    C. Start removing the gloves.
    D. Dispose of the needle in a sharps container.

Special Collections

1. What is a non-blood specimen in the context of a phlebotomy procedure?
   A. A specimen obtained from a fingerstick
   B. A sample of saliva, urine, or stool
   C. A sample of tissue taken from the patient
   D. Blood is drawn from a peripheral vein

2. Which type of skin preparation is required before collecting a urine specimen?
   A. Swabbing the area with an alcohol wipe
   B. Washing hands thoroughly with soap and water
   C. Cleaning the area with a betadine solution
   D. No special skin preparation is required

3. Why is volume essential when collecting a urine specimen?
   A. The color of the urine changes based on the volume
   B. The volume of urine can indicate kidney function
   C. A sufficient volume is required to perform the necessary tests
   D. The volume of urine indicates the level of hydration

4. What type of non-blood specimen is typically collected for a stool culture?
   A. Saliva
   B. Urine
   C. Sweat
   D. Stool

5. Which non-blood specimens might be collected to check for strep throat?
   A. Saliva
   B. Urine
   C. Throat swab
   D. Stool

6. What type of skin preparation is needed before a sweat test?
   A. Cleaning the skin with an alcohol wipe
   B. Applying a powder to absorb sweat
   C. Applying a sweat-inducing agent to the skin
   D. No preparation is needed

7. What volume of urine is typically needed for a routine urinalysis?
   A. 10 ml
   B. 25 ml
   C. 50 ml
   D. 100 ml

8. Which of the following might indicate the need for a sputum (a type of non-blood specimen) culture?
   A. Symptoms of a urinary tract infection
   B. Symptoms of a throat infection
   C. Symptoms of a lower respiratory infection
   D. Symptoms of a gastrointestinal infection

9. How should the skin be prepared before a venipuncture?
    A. By applying a warm compress
    B. By cleaning the area with an antiseptic wipe
    C. By applying a topical anesthetic
    D. By marking the vein with a skin marker

10. What blood volume is typically required for a complete blood count (CBC)?
    A. 2 ml
    B. 5 ml
    C. 10 ml
    D. 20 ml

11. What type of non-blood specimen might be collected to test for a urinary tract infection?
    A. Saliva
    B. Urine
    C. Sweat
    D. Stool

12. Why is volume crucial when collecting a blood specimen?
    A. Larger volumes allow for more accurate test results
    B. Blood volume can indicate hydration status
    C. Sufficient volume is needed to perform necessary tests
    D. Blood volume affects the color and viscosity of the sample

13. How should the skin be prepared before collecting a stool sample?
    A. Clean the area with soap and water
    B. Swab the area with an alcohol wipe
    C. No specific preparation is needed
    D. Apply an antiseptic solution to the area

14. Which non-blood specimens could be collected to diagnose a bacterial infection in the intestines?
    A. Saliva
    B. Urine
    C. Sweat
    D. Stool

15. How much saliva is usually needed for a saliva hormone test?
    A. 1 ml
    B. 2 ml
    C. 5 ml
    D. 10 ml

16. How should the skin be prepared before collecting a sweat specimen for a sweat chloride test?
    A. Clean with an alcohol wipe
    B. Apply a warm compress
    C. No specific preparation is required
    D. Clean with soap and water

17. What is a critical consideration when collecting a 24-hour urine specimen?
    A. The patient should avoid drinking fluids during the collection period
    B. The entire volume of urine passed during the 24 hours must be collected
    C. The sample should be kept at room temperature
    D. The patient should fast during the collection period

18. Why is it crucial to accurately measure and record the volume of a 24-hour urine collection?
   A. To calculate the concentration of certain substances in the urine
   B. To assess the patient's hydration status
   C. To determine the patient's renal function
   D. All of the above

19. How should the skin be prepared before collecting a nasopharyngeal swab for influenza testing?
   A. Clean with an alcohol wipe
   B. No specific preparation is required
   C. Clean with soap and water
   D. Apply an antiseptic solution

20. Why might a healthcare professional collect a sputum specimen rather than a throat swab when testing for certain respiratory infections?
   A. Sputum samples are easier to collect
   B. Sputum samples can provide more accurate results for lower respiratory infections
   C. Sputum samples can be used to test for a broader range of infections
   D. All of the above

21. When collecting a throat swab to test for strep throat, what part of the throat should be swabbed?
   A. The roof of the mouth
   B. The back of the tongue
   C. The tonsils or back of the throat
   D. The uvula

22. Why is it essential to follow specific skin preparation procedures before collecting a blood specimen for a blood culture?
   A. To minimize patient discomfort
   B. To reduce the risk of contamination by skin bacteria
   C. To improve the accuracy of the test results
   D. All of the above

23. Which of the following statements about collecting a blood specimen for glucose testing is correct?
   A. The patient should be fasting for at least 8 hours
   B. The patient should consume a high-sugar meal before the test
   C. The timing of the collection does not matter
   D. The patient should not drink water before the test

24. Why might a healthcare professional ask patients for a "first-morning" urine sample?
   A. Because urine is more concentrated in the morning
   B. Because it's easier to collect
   C. Because it reduces the risk of contamination
   D. Because it's more comfortable for the patient

25. How should a blood specimen be handled after collection to ensure accurate potassium testing?
   A. The sample should be chilled immediately
   B. The sample should be kept at room temperature
   C. The sample should be mixed gently to prevent hemolysis
   D. All of the above

Processing

1. What is the primary purpose of maintaining a chain of custody for a specimen?
   A. To document the collection and transportation process
   B. To protect patient confidentiality
   C. To verify the accuracy of the test results
   D. All of the above

2. What is the first step in the disposal process of a biological specimen?
   A. Disinfection
   B. Incineration
   C. Decontamination
   D. Autoclaving

3. What is the primary purpose of centrifugation in a clinical laboratory?
   A. To separate the components of a specimen
   B. To kill microorganisms in the specimen
   C. To increase the volume of the specimen
   D. To create a homogeneous solution

4. What is the first step in retrieving a patient's lab results in a laboratory information system (LIS)?
   A. Entering the patient's full name
   B. Entering the patient's unique ID or accession number
   C. Searching for the patient's date of birth
   D. Contacting the healthcare provider

5. What information is generally NOT included in the chain of custody documentation?
   A. patient's social security number
   B. the name of the person collecting the specimen
   C. Date and time of specimen collection
   D. Any handling and transfer activities

6. How should temperature-sensitive specimens be stored before analysis?
   A. In a standard refrigerator
   B. At room temperature
   C. In a temperature-controlled environment, as required by the specific test
   D. In a freezer

7. What is the most common method for disposing of used sharps in a clinical laboratory?
   A. Placing in a biohazard bag
   B. Putting in a puncture-resistant sharps container
   C. Wrapping in paper and place in the regular trash
   D. Washing and reusing

8. Why is it important to balance the load in a centrifuge before the operation?
   A. To prevent damage to the centrifuge
   B. To ensure even separation of the specimen components
   C. To reduce the risk of specimen spillage
   D. All of the above

9. How are critical lab values typically flagged in a laboratory information system (LIS)?
   A. By a manual review by a lab technician
   B. By an automated alert system
   C. By a notification sent to the healthcare provider
   D. By highlighting the result of the report

10. What is the most effective way to prevent specimen identification errors when handling a specimen?
    A. Double-checking the patient's identification
    B. Labeling the specimen in the presence of the patient
    C. Using barcoded labels
    D. All of the above

11. What is the main reason for using a particular chain of custody form when collecting a legal drug screen?
    A. To ensure accurate results
    B. To track the specimen from collection to testing
    C. To ensure the specimen has not been tampered with
    D. All of the above

12. How should specimens be transported to maintain integrity?
    A. In a single biohazard bag
    B. In a sturdy, leak-proof container
    C. In a temperature-appropriate environment
    D. B and C

13. What is the centrifuge's function in a laboratory setting?
    A. To mix reagents
    B. Separate particles from a solution according to size, shape, density, and viscosity.
    C. To heat samples
    D. To measure the volume of a sample

14. Which data would you most likely input into a laboratory information system (LIS)?
    A. patient's contact information
    B. Patient's health history
    C. Patient's lab test orders and results
    D. All of the above

15. A blood sample for a legal blood alcohol level should be collected in which tube type?
    A. A blue-top tube
    B. A red-top tube
    C. A grey-top tube
    D. A purple-top tube

16. If a blood culture specimen is collected, what additional action must be taken in the LIS?
    A. The specimen must be flagged for urgent processing.
    B. The specimen must be marked as biohazardous.
    C. The collection time must be recorded.
    D. The specimen must be tagged for discard after testing.

17. What is the purpose of centrifuging a blood sample?
    A. To separate the blood cells from the plasma or serum.
    B. To eliminate bacteria from the blood.
    C. To warm up the blood before testing.
    D. Mix the blood with the additives in the tube.

18. What information should be included when labeling a specimen?
    A. patient's full name and date of birth.
    B. Date and time of collection.
    C. type of specimen.
    D. All of the above.

19. What type of specimen requires storage at body temperature?
   A. Stool specimen.
   B. Semen specimen.
   C. Blood specimen.
   D. Urine specimen.

20. In a laboratory, where should hazardous waste be disposed of?
   A. Regular trash bin.
   B. Sink or drain.
   C. Designated hazardous waste container.
   D. Sharps container.

21. Which information system is primarily used for managing test orders and results in a laboratory?
   A. Electronic Health Record (EHR)
   B. Laboratory Information System (LIS)
   C. Radiology Information System (RIS)
   D. Hospital Information System (HIS)

22. What should you do if a specimen tube needs to be filled to the correct volume?
   A. Use it any way
   B. Discard the tube and collect a new specimen
   C. Fill the tube with saline to reach the correct volume
   D. Store the tube upside down

23. When handling laboratory specimens, what is the most effective way to prevent the spread of infections?
   A. Washing hands after removing gloves
   B. Using personal protective equipment (PPE)
   C. Following standard precautions at all times
   D. All of the above

24. How should a sharps container be disposed of when it's complete?
   A. Placed in the regular trash
   B. Emptied and reused
   C. Sealed and placed in a biohazard waste disposal container
   D. Sent for recycling

25. Why is it essential to follow HIPAA regulations in a clinical laboratory?
   A. To protect patient safety
   B. To prevent litigation
   C. To ensure patient privacy
   D. All of the above

ANSWER WITH EXPLANATION

Safety and Compliance

1. Answer: **B.** Employee safety.

   Reason: OSHA, or the Occupational Safety and Health Administration, is a federal agency responsible for ensuring employees' safe and healthy working conditions.

2. Answer: **B.** HIPAA

   Reason: The Health Insurance Portability and Accountability Act (HIPAA) primarily addresses patient privacy and the confidentiality of medical records.

3. Answer: **D.** Blood pressure cuff

   Reason: A blood pressure cuff is not sharp and cannot puncture or cut the skin.

4. Answer: **D.** Stethoscope

   Reason: While a stethoscope is a standard tool in healthcare, it does not provide a barrier against potential infectious material and thus is not considered personal protective equipment (PPE).

5. Answer: **C.** 20 seconds

   Reason: According to the CDC, washing hands with soap and water for at least 20 seconds is crucial for preventing the spread of germs and infection.

6. Answer: **B.** Wash the area with soap and water, then report the incident.

   Reason: In case of exposure, immediate area cleaning is necessary, followed by reporting the incident for further medical evaluation and treatment.

7. Answer: **A.** To ensure accurate and reliable test results.

   Reason: Quality control measures are used in a laboratory setting to maintain the accuracy and reliability of test results, ensuring patient safety.

8. Answer: **C.** Sharps container

   Reason: Contaminated needles and other sharp items should be disposed of in a sharps container to prevent needlestick injuries and potential exposure to pathogens.

9. Answer: **C.** Wash hands

   Reason: Hand hygiene is crucial in preventing the spread of infections; washing hands after removing gloves minimizes the risk of contamination.

10. Answer: **C.** Both A and B

   Reason: Infection control aims to protect healthcare professionals and patients from potential infections.

11. Answer: **A.** To promote high standards of practice.

   Reason: Ethical standards are primarily in place to promote high-quality care and professionalism in healthcare.

12. Answer: **D.** Store patient information securely and disclose it to authorized personnel.

   Reason: HIPAA regulations require that patient information be kept confidential and only be shared with authorized personnel.

13. Answer: **C.** Eating and drinking in the phlebotomy lab.

   Reason: Eating and drinking in areas with potential exposure to bloodborne pathogens are strictly against OSHA guidelines.

14. Answer: **C.** Dispose of it in a designated sharps container.

   Reason: Contaminated sharps should be immediately disposed of in designated sharps containers to prevent accidental injuries and infections.

15. Answer: **D.** Follow the facility's spill cleanup procedures.

   Reason: Chemical spills pose a risk to safety and health and should be cleaned up immediately following the facility's standard spill cleanup procedures, as mandated by OSHA.

16. Answer: **B.** Clean the exposed area and report the incident.

    Reason: In case of an exposure incident, the first step is to clean the exposed area immediately and then report the incident for proper evaluation and follow-up.

17. Answer: **C.** Washing for at least 20 seconds

    Reason: The time spent washing hands is one of the most critical factors in effectively reducing the number of germs and microbes. According to CDC guidelines, hands should be scrubbed for at least 20 seconds.

18. Answer: **C.** When the procedure does not involve blood or body fluids

    Reason: PPE is required when there is potential exposure to blood or other body fluids. PPE might be unnecessary if a system does not include exposure to these.

19. Answer: **B.** Ensuring that specimens are collected, stored, and handled correctly

    Reason: Quality control in phlebotomy is primarily focused on ensuring the integrity of samples by maintaining proper collection, handling, and storage procedures.

20. Answer: **C.** Controlling the exposure of healthcare workers to potentially infectious materials

    Reason: In healthcare, exposure control reduces healthcare workers' risk of exposure to bloodborne pathogens or other potentially infectious materials.

Patient Preparation

1. Answer: **C.** Use clear, understandable language and show empathy.

    Reason: Rapport is best established by maintaining professional boundaries while demonstrating empathy and understanding, which includes using clear language that patients can understand.

2. Answer: **B.** Obtain informed consent.

    Reason: The patient's informed consent should be obtained before any medical procedure, including phlebotomy. This includes explaining the process, its purpose, and any potential risks.

3. Answer: **C.** A special consideration.

    Reason: Fear of needles is a common concern for many patients. As such, it should be considered a special consideration requiring additional communication and reassurance.

4. Answer: **B.** The size, condition, and location of the vein.

    Reason: The selection of a vein for venipuncture should be based on its size, condition (such as whether it's visible or palpable), and location, as these factors can affect the ease and success of the blood draw.

5. Answer: **B.** "Start urinating in the toilet, then collect mid-stream."

    Reason: A "clean-catch" urine specimen, which helps avoid contamination, typically involves starting the urine flow into the toilet, then collecting the mid-stream flow in a specimen cup.

6. Answer: **B.** It can impact the accuracy of the test results.

    Reason: Some tests require precise timing, such as measuring levels of substances that fluctuate throughout the day (e.g., cortisol) or those that need to be done at specific times after a meal or medication dose.

7. Answer: **C.** Just before the procedure.

    Reason: Informing the patient about the purpose of the blood draw before the procedure helps ensure informed consent and promotes understanding and cooperation.

8. Answer: **C.** A special consideration.

    Reason: A history of syncope (fainting) during blood draws a special consideration that may require the phlebotomist to take extra precautions, such as having the patient lie down during the procedure.

9. Answer: **D.** It can increase the risk of lymphedema.

    Reason: Following a mastectomy, especially if lymph nodes were removed, drawing blood from the arm on the same side can increase the risk of lymphedema, which causes swelling due to a blockage in the lymphatic system.

10. Answer: **A.** A patient who has never given a stool sample before.

    Reason: Patients who have never given a stool sample before may not know how to collect the model correctly, including how much is needed and how to avoid contamination.

11. Answer: **A.** Just before the procedure.

Reason: Communicating the purpose of the procedure just before it begins is an essential part of obtaining informed consent and setting the patient's expectations.

12. Answer: **C.** Respect the patient's decision and notify the appropriate healthcare provider.

Reason: Patients have the right to refuse medical procedures. The healthcare provider should be informed so they can discuss the implications with the patient and explore alternatives if necessary.

13. Answer: **D.** By applying a topical anesthetic and providing reassurance.

Reason: Patients with needle phobia may benefit from measures to reduce pain, such as topical anesthetics, reassurance, and other anxiety-reducing techniques.

14. Answer: **B.** The fingertip.

Reason: In adults and older children, the recommended site for capillary blood collection is typically the fingertip, as it's less painful and easier to access than other areas.

15. Answer: **A.** Less than 1 minute.

Reason: Leaving a tourniquet on for more than 1 minute can affect test results, cause patient discomfort, and increase the risk of hemolysis.

16. Answer: **B.** Ask the patient to breathe deeply and slowly.

Reason: If a patient feels dizzy, the phlebotomist should stop the procedure, make sure the patient is safe (e.g., seated or lying down), and advise the patient to breathe deeply and slowly. If the dizziness persists, medical assistance should be sought.

17. Answer: **A.** The patient must be fasting.

Reason: The patient should be fasting for a GTT to ensure accurate results. The phlebotomist will then draw blood at specific intervals after the patient consumes a glucose drink.

18. Answer: **C.** Immediately remove the needle and lower the patient's head.

Reason: If a patient faints during a venipuncture, the phlebotomist should immediately remove the needle (to prevent injury) and lower the patient's head (to improve blood flow). After ensuring the patient is safe, the phlebotomist should seek medical assistance.

19. Answer: **B.** The side of the heel.

Reason: The recommended side for a heel stick on an infant is the medial or lateral plantar surface (the side of the heel). The central area of the heel should be avoided due to the risk of injuring the bone.

20. Answer: **B.** To ensure the correct patient is being tested.

Reason: Correct patient identification is a critical first step in any medical procedure, including phlebotomy. It helps prevent medical errors by ensuring the correct patient receives the appropriate test or treatment.

21. Answer: **A.** First-morning urine.

Reason: The first-morning urine is typically used for pregnancy testing because it is more concentrated and likely to contain higher hormone levels (hCG), especially in early pregnancy.

22. Answer: **D.** Veins may be more fragile and prone to bruising.

Reason: In geriatric patients, skin and veins may be more delicate, requiring gentle handling to avoid bruising or injury.

23. Answer: **A.** Before and after each patient contact.

Reason: Hand hygiene is essential to prevent the spread of infection. A phlebotomist should wash their hands before and after each patient contact, after removing gloves, and when their hands are visibly soiled.

24. Answer: **B.** Respect the patient's decision, inform the patient's healthcare provider, and document the incident.

Reason: A patient can refuse treatment, including blood draws. If a patient refuses, the phlebotomist should respect the patient's decision, inform the patient's healthcare provider, and document the incident.

25. Answer: **B.** By using a safety-engineered needle and following proper disposal procedures.

Reason: To prevent needlestick injuries, a phlebotomist should use a safety-engineered needle and follow the proper disposal procedures. This usually involves placing used needles in a designated sharps container without recapping. Washing hands is also crucial but doesn't directly prevent needlestick injuries.

Routine Blood Collections

1. Answer: **C.** Needle and holder

    Reason: Before beginning the venipuncture procedure, the phlebotomist should assemble the needle and holder to ensure they are ready when needed.

2. Answer: **D.** Blue, red, lavender, green

    Reason: The correct order of draw minimizes the chance of cross-contamination of additives between tubes, and it is typically as follows: blood culture bottles or tubes, coagulation tube (blue), serum tubes with or without clot activator/gel (red), heparin tubes (green), EDTA tubes (lavender), and lastly glucose tubes (gray).

3. Answer: **D.** Isopropyl alcohol

    Reason: Isopropyl alcohol is the most commonly used antiseptic for routine venipuncture because it's effective against bacteria present on the skin.

4. Answer: **A.** Patient's full name, date of birth, date and time of collection, and phlebotomist's initials

    Reason: Labeling a specimen accurately is crucial to patient safety. The label should include the patient's full name, date of birth, date and time of collection, and the phlebotomist's initials.

5. Answer: **B.** Apply pressure to the venipuncture site.

    Reason: After removing the needle, the first step in post-procedure care is to apply pressure to the venipuncture site to prevent bleeding and bruising.

6. Answer: **D.** After disposing of the used needle and holder in a sharps container.

    Reason: The phlebotomist should keep their gloves on until all patient contact has ended and all equipment used for the draw, including the needle, has been safely disposed of.

7. Answer: **B.** To prevent cross-contamination of additives between tubes.

    Reason: The correct order of draw is essential to prevent cross-contamination of additives between tubes, which could compromise the accuracy of the test results.

8. Answer: **A.** 15-30 degrees.

    Reason: The needle should be inserted at an angle of 15-30 degrees during venipuncture to avoid going through the vein or causing trauma to the area.

9. Answer: **C.** After blood starts to flow into the tube.

    Reason: The tourniquet should be released after blood flows into the tube and before removing the needle. This helps to minimize patient discomfort and vein damage.

10. Answer: **A.** Mix the blood with the additives in the tube.

    Reason: Tubes should be inverted after collection to ensure proper blood mixing with the additives in the tube.

11. Answer: **C.** In a sharps container

    Reason: Used sharps (needles, lancets, etc.) should always be disposed of in a sharps container to prevent accidental injuries and spreading infection.

12. Answer: **A.** To protect the phlebotomist from exposure to blood and other body fluids

    Reason: PPE, such as gloves and lab coats, protects healthcare workers from exposure to potential pathogens found in blood and other body fluids.

13. Answer: **B.** Immediately wash the area with soap and water

    Reason: The first action after a needlestick injury is to clean the area with soap and water to reduce the risk of infection. After this, the incident should be reported to a supervisor for further action.

14. Answer: **D.** All of the above

    Reason: The lid should always be placed on the specimen tube after collection to prevent spillage, evaporation, and exposure to air, all of which can affect the quality of the specimen and the accuracy of test results.

15. Answer: **B.** To facilitate blood flow

    Reason: The patient's arm should be positioned downward to use gravity to help facilitate blood flow, making the collection process easier and more efficient.

16. Answer: **B.** Immediately remove the needle, apply pressure to the site, and position the patient in a way to restore blood flow to the brain.

Reason: Safety is a priority. In the case of a patient fainting, the procedure should be immediately halted. The needle must be removed carefully, and pressure applied to prevent excessive bleeding. The patient should be positioned appropriately to restore blood flow to the brain, generally laying flat or with feet elevated if possible.

17. Answer: **B.** The right arm

Reason: Blood should not be drawn from an arm on the same side as a mastectomy without permission from the patient's physician. The procedure could cause complications such as lymphedema. Therefore, in this case, the right arm should be used for the blood draw.

18. Answer: **C.** Inverting the tube gently several times

Reason: The proper way to mix a blood sample with an anticoagulant in a collection tube is by gently inverting the line several times. Vigorous shaking can lead to hemolysis, damaging the cells and potentially impacting the test results.

19. Answer: **B.** CBC tube, electrolyte panel tube, coagulation tube

Reason: The standard order of draw is as follows: blood culture tubes (if needed), coagulation tubes (light blue), serum tubes with or without clot activator and with or without gel (red, gold, speckled), heparin tubes with or without gel plasma separator (light/dark green), EDTA tubes (lavender), and lastly, fluoride tubes (gray). In this case, the CBC (usually lavender), electrolyte panel (typically green or gold), and coagulation test (light blue) should follow this order.

20. Answer: **D.** All of the above.

Reason: All the mentioned techniques can enhance vein visibility and palpability. The method chosen depends on the situation and the patient's condition. If a suitable vein is still not found, you may need to select a different venipuncture site or ask for assistance from a colleague.

21. Answer: **D.** Isopropyl alcohol

Reason: Isopropyl alcohol is the most commonly used antiseptic for routine venipuncture because of its fast and effective antimicrobial properties. Other agents can be used, but they may require a longer drying time or be contraindicated for certain patients.

22. Answer: **D.** The phlebotomist should identify the patient by their full name and date of birth.

Reason: Proper patient identification, usually through confirming the patient's full name and date of birth, is crucial to ensuring patient safety and the accuracy of test results. Relying on the patient's bed number or a missing ID band is not a reliable form of identification.

23. Answer: **B.** Upward

Reason: When performing a venipuncture, the bevel of the needle should face upward. This allows for a smoother insertion, minimizing discomfort for the patient and reducing the risk of puncturing through the other side of the vein.

24. Answer: **C.** Stop the procedure, inform the patient's healthcare provider, and document the incident.

Reason: Patient consent is critical for any procedure, including phlebotomy. If a patient refuses a procedure, the phlebotomist should stop immediately, inform the healthcare provider, and document the refusal and any other relevant information.

25. Answer: **A.** Remove the tourniquet.

Reason: The tourniquet should be removed as soon as blood flow is established and the tubes begin to fill. This minimizes potential discomfort for the patient and reduces the risk of hemoconcentration or hematoma formation. The needle disposal, bandage application, and glove removal follow afterward.

Special Collections

1. Answer: **B.** A sample of saliva, urine, or stool

   Reason: Non-blood specimens in a phlebotomy context refer to body fluids other than blood, such as saliva, urine, and stool. These samples can provide valuable diagnostic information depending on the tests the physician orders.

2. Answer: **B.** Washing hands thoroughly with soap and water

   Reason: Before collecting a urine specimen, the patient should wash their hands thoroughly with soap and water. This reduces the likelihood of the sample being contaminated with bacteria from the hands.

3. Answer: **C.** A sufficient volume is required to perform the necessary tests

   Reason: It's essential to manage enough volume to conduct the ordered tests when collecting a urine specimen. Inadequate volume may not allow for complete testing, leading to potential inaccuracies or the need for additional collections.

4. Answer: **D.** Stool

   Reason: A stool culture is a laboratory test that checks for any bacteria or other organisms in the stool that can cause disease. It's commonly used to identify a foodborne illness or infection.

5. Answer: **C.** Throat swab

   Reason: A throat swab is often used to check for a streptococcus (strep) infection in the throat. The sample is obtained by swabbing the back of the throat and tonsils to get cells to test for the bacteria.

6. Answer: **C.** Applying a sweat-inducing agent to the skin

   Reason: A sweat-inducing agent is often applied to the skin before a sweat test. This helps ensure enough sweat is produced for the test, which measures chloride levels in work and helps diagnose conditions like cystic fibrosis.

7. Answer: **C.** 50 ml

   Reason: A routine urinalysis typically requires about 50 ml of urine. This volume allows for a variety of tests to be performed, including physical, chemical, and microscopic examinations.

8. Answer: **C.** Symptoms of a lower respiratory infection

   Reason: A sputum culture is often ordered when a patient has symptoms of a lower respiratory tract infection, such as a persistent cough, chest pain, or difficulty breathing. This test can identify the presence of bacteria, fungi, or viruses in the sputum that might be causing the infection.

9. Answer: **B.** By cleaning the area with an antiseptic wipe

   Reason: Before a venipuncture, the skin should be prepared by cleaning the area with an antiseptic wipe. This helps prevent infection by killing any bacteria on the skin's surface.

10. Answer: **A.** 2 ml

    Reason: A typical complete blood count (CBC) requires about 2 ml. This volume is usually sufficient to allow for the variety of tests included in a CBC, such as measuring the levels of different types of blood cells.

11. Answer: **B.** Urine

    Reason: A urine specimen is typically collected to test for a urinary tract infection. The sample can be examined under a microscope, cultured to grow any bacteria present, and experimented with chemical strips to detect signs of infection.

12. Answer: **C.** Sufficient volume is needed to perform necessary tests

    Reason: When collecting a blood specimen, collecting a sufficient volume is essential to perform the required tests. An adequate volume may prevent complete testing and could lead to inaccuracies or the need for additional collections.

13. Answer: **C.** No specific preparation is needed

    Reason: Generally, no specific skin preparation is needed before collecting a stool sample. However, the model should be collected in a clean, dry container to avoid contamination.

14. Answer: **D.** Stool

    Reason: A stool sample can diagnose a bacterial infection in the intestines. The model is cultured in a lab to identify the presence and type of bacteria.

15. Answer: **B.** 2 ml

   Reason: Around 2 ml of saliva is needed for most saliva hormone tests. The sample is then analyzed in a laboratory to measure hormone levels.

16. Answer: **C.** No specific preparation is required

   Reason: The area of skin where the sweat will be collected does not need any special preparation before a sweat chloride test, often used to diagnose cystic fibrosis. The test involves applying a substance that stimulates sweating and then collecting the sweat for analysis.

17. Answer: **B.** The entire volume of urine passed during the 24 hours must be collected

   Reason: When a 24-hour urine specimen is requested, all urine passed during the 24 hours must be collected. This provides a comprehensive overview of the substances excreted in the urine, allowing for a more accurate diagnosis.

18. Answer: **D.** All of the above

   Reason: Measuring and recording a 24-hour urine collection volume is crucial for various reasons. It allows healthcare professionals to calculate the concentration of specific substances in the urine, assess the patient's hydration status, and determine their renal function.

19. Answer: **B.** No specific preparation is required

   Reason: No specific skin preparation is required before collecting a nasopharyngeal swab for influenza testing. The swab is inserted into the nostril and back to the nasopharynx, ordering a sample of cells and secretions.

20. Answer: **B.** Sputum samples can provide more accurate results for lower respiratory infections

   Reason: While throat swabs can be used to test for some respiratory infections, a sputum sample may provide more accurate results for infections in the lower respiratory tract, such as pneumonia or tuberculosis. This is because the sputum is deep inside the lungs, where these infections typically occur.

21. Answer: **C.** The tonsils or back of the throat

   Reason: When collecting a throat swab to test for strep throat, the swab should be gently rubbed over the tonsils or back of the throat. This is where the streptococcal bacteria, if present, are likely to be found.

22. Answer: **D.** All of the above

   Reason: It is essential to follow specific skin preparation procedures before collecting a blood specimen for a blood culture to minimize patient discomfort, reduce the risk of contamination by skin bacteria, and improve the accuracy of the test results.

23. Answer: **A.** The patient should be fasting for at least 8 hours

   Reason: When collecting a blood specimen for glucose testing, the patient should have been fasting for at least 8 hours to ensure the results are not influenced by recent food or drink intake.

24. Answer: **A.** Because urine is more concentrated in the morning

   Reason: A "first-morning" urine sample is often requested because urine is more concentrated after a night's sleep. This higher concentration can make it easier to detect specific substances, such as hormones or metabolites, that might be present in smaller amounts in less concentrated urine.

25. Answer: **C.** The sample should be mixed gently to prevent hemolysis

   Reason: The model should be combined gently after collecting a blood specimen for potassium testing. Aggressive mixing or shaking can cause hemolysis or breaking of the red blood cells, releasing potassium into the serum and leading to falsely elevated results.

Processing

1. Answer: **D.** All of the above

   Reason: A chain of custody is used to document the collection, handling, and storage process of a specimen, protect patient confidentiality, and verify the accuracy of test results.

2. Answer: **C.** Decontamination

   Reason: Decontamination is the first step in safely disposing of biological specimens to ensure that all biohazardous materials are removed.

3. Answer: **A.** To separate the components of a specimen

   Reason: Centrifugation is used to separate the members of a model based on their densities.

4. Answer: **B.** Entering the patient's unique ID or accession number

   Reason: The patient's unique ID or accession number is the primary identifier in a laboratory information system (LIS).

5. Answer: **A.** Patient's social security number

   Reason: The patient's social security number is usually not included in the chain of custody documentation to protect patient confidentiality.

6. Answer: **C.** In a temperature-controlled environment, as required by the specific test

   Reason: Different specimens may require different storage conditions. Temperature-sensitive samples should be stored in a temperature-controlled environment for the specific test.

7. Answer: **B.** Putting in a puncture-resistant sharps container

   Reason: Used sharps should be disposed of in a puncture-resistant sharps container to prevent injury and potential infection.

8. Answer: **D.** All of the above

   Reason: It's essential to balance the load in a centrifuge to prevent damage to the machine, ensure even separation of the specimen components, and reduce the risk of specimen spillage.

9. Answer: **B.** By an automated alert system

   Reason: Critical lab values are typically flagged in a LIS by an automated alert system, which helps ensure that these critical results are quickly recognized and acted upon.

10. Answer: **D.** All of the above

    Reason: The most effective way to prevent specimen identification errors is to use multiple strategies, including double-checking the patient's identification, labeling the specimen in the patient's presence, and using barcoded labels.

11. Answer: **D.** All of the above

    Reason: Chain of custody forms track the specimen from collection to testing, ensure accurate results, and ensure the model hasn't been tampered with.

12. Answer: **D.** B and C

    Reason: To maintain their integrity, specimens should be transported in a sturdy, leak-proof container and in a temperature-appropriate environment.

13. Answer: **B.** Separate particles from a solution according to size, shape, density, and viscosity.

    Reason: A centrifuge is used in a laboratory setting to separate particles from a solution based on size, shape, density, and viscosity.

14. Answer: **C.** Patient's lab test orders and results

    Reason: While a LIS might contain a wide range of data, its primary purpose is to manage data related to a patient's lab test orders and results.

15. Answer: **C.** A grey-top tube

    Reason: A grey-top tube contains sodium fluoride and potassium oxalate. Sodium fluoride is a preservative that prevents the breakdown of glucose, while potassium oxalate is an anticoagulant.

16. Answer: **C.** The collection time must be recorded.

    Reason: The collection time for blood culture specimens is fundamental because it helps track the growth of bacteria or other microorganisms in the blood over time.

17. Answer: **A.** To separate the blood cells from the plasma or serum.

    Reason: Centrifugation separates the various components of blood based on their densities. This allows for more accurate testing and analysis of the different parts.

18. Answer: **D.** All of the above.

Reason: All the above information is necessary to correctly identify and track the specimen. Any information that needs to be included could lead to errors or mix-ups.

19. Answer: **B.** Semen specimen.

Reason: Semen specimens for fertility studies must be kept at body temperature to maintain the viability of the sperm.

20. Answer: **C.** Designated hazardous waste container.

Reason: Hazardous waste must be disposed of in a designated container to ensure safety and compliance with waste disposal regulations.

21. Answer: **B.** Laboratory Information System (LIS)

Reason: A Laboratory Information System (LIS) is designed to manage and store data from laboratory test orders and results. It is specialized in laboratory workflows and procedures.

22. Answer: **B.** Discard the tube and collect a new specimen

Reason: The volume of the model is critical for accurate testing. If a tube is not filled with the correct book, a new model should be collected to ensure accurate test results.

23. Answer: **D.** All of the above

Reason: All of these methods are crucial for preventing the spread of infections when handling laboratory specimens.

24. Answer: **C.** Sealed and placed in a biohazard waste disposal container

Reason: Sharps containers, when complete, should be sealed and placed in a biohazard waste disposal container for proper treatment and disposal.

25. Answer: **D.** All of the above

Reason: HIPAA regulations aim to ensure patient safety, prevent litigation, and maintain patient privacy by setting standards for handling patient health information. Failure to adhere to these standards can lead to severe penalties.

CONCLUSION

Phlebotomy is an integral part of the healthcare system, playing a crucial role in the diagnosis, treatment, and overall understanding of patient health. This guide was designed to provide a comprehensive overview of the elements required for the National Health career Association (NHA) phlebotomy exam and to serve as a valuable resource for aspiring phlebotomists.

Throughout the chapters, we have delved into the essential aspects of phlebotomy, including the foundational knowledge of human anatomy, particularly the circulatory system, to the technical skills required for various blood collection techniques. The responsibilities and ethical standards required of a phlebotomist were thoroughly examined to ensure readers are prepared for their multifaceted role.

From patient interactions and communication strategies to the details of specimen collection, handling, and legal standards, the importance of maintaining patient safety and comfort while ensuring the accuracy and quality of the results has been emphasized.

Additionally, this guide incorporated a range of test practice materials, including frequently asked and multiple-choice questions designed to emulate the structure of the NHA phlebotomy exam. The glossary provided at the end of the guide is a quick reference point for critical terms and concepts.

The journey toward becoming a certified phlebotomist is challenging but rewarding. We hope the insights and information provided in this guide will assist you in your studies and enhance your understanding of phlebotomy. We wish you the best of luck on your NHA phlebotomy exam and future career as a phlebotomist. Your dedication to this field will undoubtedly contribute to enhancing patient care and advancing the healthcare industry.

SPECIAL BONUS

D ear reader, I would be grateful if you would take a minute of your time and post a review on AMAZON to let other users know how this experience was and what you liked most about the book.
Also, I have recently decided to offer bonuses to all our readers. Yes, I want to provide you with the assistance that will help you with your study you will receive:

- **MP3 audio files** ready to rock on your drive, at the gym, wherever you choose!
- **A digital copy** of this book, always at your fingertips.
- **A glossary** of critical terms to review wherever, whenever.
- **20 case studies** that put you right into the action!
- A PDF copy of the book **"Medical Terms for Healthcare Professions"**, your essential sidekick.
- **+600 flashcards <u>with pictures</u>** to maximize your learning and cut down your study time!

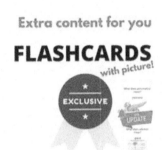

Note. FLASHCARDS ARE READY TO USE FOR FREE online or offline! You can track your progress and conveniently and interactively memorize the most important terms and concepts! Download to your device: **Anki APP or Anki Droid**, or enter the web page and register free of charge. Then import the files we have given you as a gift and use the flashcards whenever and wherever you want to study and track your progress.

Below you will find a **QR CODE** that will give you direct access to this bonus (file to download directly to your device) without having to subscribe to any mailing list or leave your personal information.

I hope you will appreciate it.

To communicate with us directly, (or if you have any problem with download of extra content) please, write to us at **info.testbookreader@gmail.com**

We are waiting for your feedback on amazon, in any case!
A cordial greeting; we wish you all the best.

Thank you!

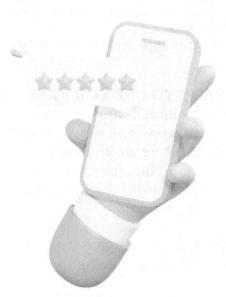

THANK YOU!

Made in the USA
Las Vegas, NV
24 February 2024

86200646R00057